# The Mental Status Examination in Neurology

## SECOND EDITION

# The Mental Status Examination in Neurology

## SECOND EDITION

## Richard L. Strub, MD

Professor of Neurology
Louisiana State University Medical Center
New Orleans, Louisiana

## F. William Black, PhD

Associate Professor of Neurology and Psychiatry
Louisiana State University Medical Center
New Orleans, Louisiana

Foreword by Norman Geschwind

F.A. DAVIS COMPANY Philadelphia

Printed in the United States of America

NOTE: As new scientific information becomes available through basic and clinical research, recommended treatments and drug therapies undergo changes. The authors and publisher have done everything possible to make this book accurate, up-to-date, and in accord with accepted standards at the time of publication. However, the reader is advised always to check product information (package inserts) for changes and new information regarding dose and contraindications before administering any drug. Caution is especially urged when using new or infrequently ordered drugs.

**Library of Congress Cataloging in Publication Data**

Strub, Richard L., 1939–
　The mental status examination in neurology.

　Includes bibliographies and index.
　1. Brain damage—Diagnosis.  2. Neuropsychological tests.  3. Neurologic examination.  I. Black, F. William.  II. Title. [DNLM: 1. Nervous System Diseases—diagnosis.  2. Neurologic Examination. WL 141 S925m]
RC387.5.S77　1985　　　　616.85'884　　　　84-23169
ISBN 0-8036-8211-5

In memory of Dr. Norman Geschwind, 1926–1984

# Foreword

The testing of mental status has a curious, not to say anomalous, position in the examination of patients. Every medical student has had the experience of being given a long and detailed outline, or an even longer booklet, containing a seemingly endless list of items. Even if he should go to the trouble of memorizing these miniature compendia, he is likely to discover that his teachers, both neurologic and psychiatric, are disinclined to be concerned with the detailed examination, and often rely, at best, on fragments. The examinations themselves seem to differ from those in other fields of medicine. The student rapidly comes to appreciate the direct relevance of rectal tenderness to the diagnosis of appendicitis or or pulsus paradoxus to pericardial effusion. The mental examination seems to him to be much more indirectly and diffusely related to diagnostic categories.

Equally striking, or even more so, is the usual lack of direct correlation between the test items and disorders of structure or physiology. Orthopnea, swollen neck veins, rales at the lung bases, cardiac enlargement, characteristic murmurs, and auricular fibrillation not only mean congestive failure, but all the findings on examination come to blend almost imperceptibly and effortlessly with knowledge of normal cardiac structures and physiology and awareness of lawful derangements in disease. This easy understanding of the relationship of abnormal findings on examination to anatomy and physiology seems to be lacking in the mental examination.

There is, however, no reason that this situation should persist. The growth of knowledge concerning disorders of the higher functions has been rapid over the past quarter century. Not only has our ability to specify anatomic systems involved in different behaviors increased, but even more important, we have come to a deeper understanding of the mechanisms underlying disordered function.

This book, therefore, represents a valuable synthesis. For the attentive reader, it will yield important advantages. Not only does it shift the emphasis to those methods of examination that have proven their worth in the clinic, but it provides wherever possible a link to known anatomic and physiologic mechanisms.

Several final comments are appropriate. There is a widespread, usually tacit but often openly expressed, view that mental examination is a long and arduous task. Most physicians have learned that although a "complete" survey of the heart, lungs, abdomen, and other structures can take hours, intimate knowledge of the examination and repeated practice enable them to obtain essential information in a very brief time. Those who have learned the mental examination and have practiced it often can equally well obtain vital information rapidly and efficiently when necessary. There is another common view that mental examination can be handed over to others. We should remember, however, that the real measure of a physician's usefulness lies in his capacity to make critical decisions when he is alone with the patient in the small hours of the night. Furthermore, unless he can screen patients effectively, he will fail to refer intelligently to others. Finally, if the ultimate decisions lie in his hands, he will fail to use adequately the opinions of his consultants unless he has a basic understanding of all aspects of his patient's problems. The newer knowledge of mental examination set forth within this book is essential not merely to the neurologist or psychiatrist, but to all physicians.

Norman Geschwind, M.D.
James Jackson Putnam Professor of Neurology
Harvard Medical School
1977

# Preface

The basic purpose and scope of this book have not changed since the first edition was published in 1977. In the intervening years, we have gained considerable additional clinical experience with the mental status examination and have standardized certain sections of the examination. The standardized items have been compared with the objective data generated from formal neuropsychologic tests. These comparisons have been very rewarding, as the mental status examination has proven to be an accurate and valid method for identifying and diagnosing organic brain disease, as well as for describing relative levels of functioning.

In this edition, we have extensively rewritten the chapters that deal with behavioral observations and the diagnostic problem of differentiating among depression, dementia, and pseudodementia. We have purposely not attempted to include extensive material pertaining to primary psychiatric symptoms; this book principally deals with cognitive changes and the more dramatic personality changes seen in organic brain disease. The purely psychiatric perspective has been amply discussed in other readily available sources.

In the first edition, we assured the reader that after reading and using the book, he or she would be able to perform a brief screening examination. It has been suggested that we provide more concrete guidelines for tailoring the examination for brief administration. Therefore, in the summary section of this edition, we have included some ways to use the examination as a screening procedure, particularly in the extremely important areas of diagnosing dementia and differentiating between organic and functional disorders.

We have updated and expanded the references in all chapters; this is particularly true in those sections in which new studies have refined the neuroanatomic and neuropsychologic aspects of cognitive functions. The section on neuropsychologic testing has been fully revised to include a survey of the most commonly used tests, to drop some tests that have fallen from general use, and to make this section more clinically relevant to both physicians and psychologists.

In general, we feel that the first edition was good and has proven its value in widespread clinical use; however, the second edition is better because we have now refined the examination and have attempted to answer the questions generated by the first edition. Hopefully, this text will prove as useful to others who are interested in neurobehavior as it has been with our students, residents, and professional colleagues.

R. L. Strub, M.D.
F. W. Black, Ph.D.

# Contents

# CHAPTER 1

# The Mental Status Examination: A Rationale and Overview

Human behavior is an extremely complex, multifaceted entity. The understanding of its disruption in brain disease is a substantial and often frustrating problem to the clinician who is faced with the tasks of diagnosis and management. Patients with organically related changes in intellectual or emotional behavior unfortunately have often fallen just outside of the limits of both psychiatry and neurology. Behavioral problems within this somewhat uncharted borderland have long been subsumed under the rubric of "the organic brain syndromes," a general term that covers any possible behavior change resulting from brain damage or dysfunction. In the latest edition of the American Psychiatric Association's *Diagnostic and Statistical Manual of Mental Disorders* (DSM-III),[1] such conditions are categorized as "organic mental disorders." The DSM-III makes a distinction between an organic brain syndrome, which refers to a general clinical constellation of behavioral signs and symptoms (e.g., delirium or dementia), and an organic mental disorder, which denotes a specific disease entity such as Alzheimer's dementia or an amnesic syndrome secondary to head trauma. The neurologic literature, however, has tended to use the term neurobehavioral disorder for such conditions.

In recent years, there has been a renewed interest in these organic syndromes. It is now possible to understand many of these conditions and to assign specific patterns of behavioral deficits to specific diseases and to damage in particular regions of the brain.

Although the study of the neurobehavioral disorders has not yet reached the stage of medical popularity of arteriosclerotic heart disease, cancer, or immunologic disorders, the magnitude and social impact of neurobehavioral disorders must not be underestimated. These disorders are very common in both hospital and office practice. Dementia, aphasia, and confusional states (delirium) are not rare conditions that medical students dutifully learn about in medical school and then fruitlessly

1

search for in clinical practice. Quite the opposite is true: these are problems that the average clinician sees every day but has typically never learned about in school. Hopefully, tomorrow's students will recognize early dementia as readily as they do acquired immune deficiency syndrome or Addison's disease. Primary organic brain disease accounts for at least 30 percent of all first admissions to psychiatric hospitals[3] and has been reported to be the third most frequent cause for hospital admission among all patients with suspected neurologic disease.[2]

For examiners to adequately understand organically based behavior change and to apply this understanding to individual clinical cases, they must utilize a systematic behavioral examination. This evaluation is the mental status examination. It is an orderly assessment of the important cognitive and emotional functions that are commonly and characteristically disturbed in patients with organic brain disease.

Because the mental status examination is not always included in a comprehensive neurologic evaluation, it is important that the clinician be able to determine when inclusion of the mental status examination is appropriate. Just as the patient with otitis externa does not routinely require an electrocardiogram, the patient with a peripheral neuropathy does not usually need a full mental status examination. Conversely, the patient who complains of memory difficulty should have a comprehensive mental status examination, just as the patient with a fever, headache, and stiff neck requires an immediate CT scan and lumbar puncture.

There are many patients for whom full mental status testing is definitely indicated. Patients with known brain lesions such as tumors, trauma, or vascular accident should have a screening mental status evaluation to document any cognitive or emotional changes. It is a sad but true commentary on the current state of neurobehavioral knowledge in medicine that subtle (and sometimes gross) deficits secondary to brain lesions are overlooked or considered inconsequential by the primary physician. Many patients with mild aphasias or memory deficits after craniotomy, increased irritability and decreased ability to concentrate after head trauma, or marked emotional lability following infectious neurologic disease are released from the hospital without recognition of these cognitive and emotional deficits. Such patients frequently become emotionally frustrated, have difficulty with social readjustment, and are unable to carry out the demands of home and vocation. Early recognition of the neurobehavioral sequelae of a known neurologic disorder helps the physician explain the totality of the patient's disability to family and employers; this prevents needless frustration on the patient's part. Such documentation is of immeasurable aid in planning social and vocational rehabilitation when indicated.

There is another large group of patients in whom mental status testing is indicated. These are patients in whom a brain lesion is suspected because of recent onset of seizures, headaches, behavior change, or head trauma. Brain tumors, subdural hematomas, small infarcts, or cerebral atrophy may be undetected on the routine neurologic examination; whereas the cognitive effects of these lesions may often be readily apparent on a complete mental status examination. Thus, the inclusion of the mental status examination as a component of the initial neurologic evaluation may significantly increase the probability of detecting neurologic disease when present and effectively ruling it out when absent. We have seen a 46-year-old man who was admitted to the infectious disease isolation unit because of fever, "jumbled" speech, and "confusion." His admitting diagnosis was "probable encephalitis." Subsequent mental status testing the morning following admission revealed an aphasia rather than a confusional state. Because the finding of aphasia is almost pathognomonic of significant left-hemisphere disease, a left carotid arteriogram was performed and a large subdural hematoma was found. With appropriate treatment (surgery), the patient had an uneventful and complete recovery. Had the correct diagnosis not been made quickly, the patient could well have died without appropriate treatment and with the incorrect diagnosis of "devastating herpes simplex encephalitis." In patients in whom the diagnosis of neurologic disease is equivocal, the mental status examination may be as specific in documenting a brain lesion and indicating its location as the elicitation of a Babinski sign.

We feel that a full mental status examination should be performed on all psychiatric patients, particularly those whose psychiatric symptoms have appeared rather acutely and are superimposed upon a life history of normal emotional functioning. Organic brain disease frequently initially presents as emotional and behavioral change and comes first to the attention of the psychiatrist or the family physician. This presentation is especially characteristic of frontal and temporal tumors, hydrocephalus, or cortical atrophy.

The most common emotional change seen in these patients is depression. Brain disease should be strongly suspected in any patient with a middle- or late-life depression that is not clearly related to a recent emotional or social crisis (i.e., adjustment disorder with depressed mood). In our clinical practice, we have seen a large number of patients who were being treated with psychotropic drugs, psychotherapy, electroshock, or long-term psychiatric hospitalization for an apparent depressive illness who have, in fact, demonstrated clear signs of primary organic disease on mental status testing and subsequent neurodiagnostic procedures (e.g., CT scan and neuropsychologic evaluation). It is far more economical, efficacious, and appropriate to spend 15 minutes during the initial interview doing a complete mental status examination than to embark upon a lengthy, expensive, and sometimes inappropriate treatment regimen.

The differentiation between psychiatric and organic disease is often difficult and is not always possible. The functionally depressed patient with psychomotor retardation may perform poorly on some aspects of the mental status examination and in this way present the picture of a pseudodementia. Other patients have elements of both organic and functional disease; for example, patients with early Alzheimer's dementia often present with significant associated depression or agitation. At times, considerable effort is required to separate the respective components even on careful examination. The mental status examination is not infallible even in the hands of an experienced examiner. The fact remains, however, that the majority of such patients with combined problems will be correctly classified if appropriate mental testing is done.

A final group of patients in whom mental status screening is extremely important consists of those who initially present or are brought in by their families with vague behavioral complaints that are difficult to clinically substantiate and quantify on standard neurologic examination.

Complaints such as memory problems, difficulties in concentration, declining interest in family or work, or various physical complaints without organic etiology should alert the clinician to the possibility of organic brain disease. The determination of the etiology of such problems involves a difficult differentiation among functional, neurologic, and other medical causes. Again, this can often be accomplished with the aid of data provided by the mental status examination.

Mental status testing must be arranged in a systematic fashion. In this sense, the examination is analogous to any comprehensive medical examination. The mental status examination does differ somewhat in that it must be performed in a hierarchical manner, beginning with the most basic function—level of consciousness—and proceeding to the more complex areas of verbal reasoning and calculating ability.

When the patient shows impaired performance on early sections of the examination, for example, in language, it will be difficult, if not impossible, for the examiner to accurately assess verbal memory (an extremely important function) or any other function that requires language. Similarly, the patient who is inattentive will miss important details during much of the higher-level testing, especially the memory and calculation items. If the mental status examination is performed in a haphazard manner without regard for the hierarchical nature of cognitive performance, erroneous conclusions will be drawn. The examination must be performed in an orderly way, with the assessment of basic processes such as the level of consciousness, attention, and vigilance first, and the higher-level functions such as abstract reasoning and special cognitive functions tested last.

The mental status examination as presented in this book may seem exceptionally detailed, and it may appear that the examination would take hours to complete in its entirety. This conception is similar to the beginning clinician's first attempts to understand the evaluation of the cranial nerves or the brachial plexus. When first learning to administer the examination, it is wise to evaluate several patients fully to gain experience in performing and interpreting all test items. With time, the examination can be completed rapidly (within 15 to 20 minutes) and will yield considerable valuable data. In Chapter 10, we have summarized the examination and indicated how it can be tailored to meet the demands of time and the particular patient.

In many cases, a brief examination will provide definitive data to allow the correct diagnosis and appropriate medical treatment. As an example of the ease of administering a meaningful examination in a brief period of time, a psychiatrist, called in the middle of the night to see a patient who was "talking out of his head," started to examine the patient's language and found that the patient was actually aphasic and not psychotic. At this point, the psychiatrist consulted with the neurologist, who admitted the patient to the neurology ward rather than to the psychiatric unit. In this case, the psychiatrist had properly evaluated the patient and averted an inappropriate type of hospitalization and treatment. We were called in to see a similar case, in which a young man had been admitted to the psychiatric service because he was answering questions inappropriately and did not make sense in conversation. This behavior had initially disturbed his parents, who had brought him to the emergency room. Upon evaluation, the patient had little, if any, comprehension of language and was producing fluent paraphasic speech (aphasia). Neurodiagnostic evaluation revealed a large hematoma in the dominant temporal lobe. His "craziness" was due to a readily apparent organic disorder, and his psychiatric hospitalization had resulted from the admitting physician's lack of recognition of the patient's actual condition. In this case, demonstration of a typical pattern of aphasia not only indicated that organic disease was present, but also strongly suggested the location of the lesion.

These clinical examples illustrate that even a brief examination in the hands of the skilled examiner can be of critical clinical importance. In other patients, however, a more comprehensive assessment will be required. The patient who is referred after a head injury requires a detailed elucidation of cognitive strengths and deficits to allow for appropriate social and vocational rehabilitation. This need for a comprehensive mental status examination is amply demonstrated in the following case. The physical medicine service requested a consultation on a 32-year-old woman who had suffered a severe basilar skull fracture several months previously and was not progressing satisfactorily in the inpatient rehabilitation program. There were also questions of "difficult" and "uncooperative" behavior. Mental status testing revealed an apathetic patient without insight or concern, who had moderately impaired attention and vigilance. Multiple significant cognitive deficits were demonstrated, including a mild general dementia, moderately impaired recent and remote memory, severely impaired new-learning ability, and a moderate to severe impairment of all higher-level cognitive functions (abstraction, calculations, and so forth). The documentation of an organic behavior change and significant cognitive deficits helped to explain both the patient's difficult ward behavior and her inability to fully participate in a demanding rehabilitation program. Her program was restructured and her goals were altered because of the limitations caused by her cognitive and behavioral deficits.

In complicated situations when extensive and quantitative data regarding cognitive and emotional functioning are required for proper patient management, consultation should be obtained from relevant ancillary professionals. These include psychologists and speech pathologists. The bedside or office mental status examination as outlined in this book is very effective for diagnosing organic disease and for evaluating major areas of deficit. By its nature, the examination is qualitative and does not offer the advantages of standardized quantitative data, which are necessary for evaluating subtle deficits, planning for comprehensive rehabilitation efforts, and assessing improvements in performance. The neuropsychologist can provide these data and additional valuable consultation when a definitive evaluation is required for whatever reason. In patients with significant communication problems, referral to the speech pathologist for comprehensive evaluation of language, possible treatment, and counseling to facilitate communication between the patient and other family members is important. Chapter 11 deals in detail with the specifics of the consultation process. Every clinician should be aware of the availability and scope of such ancillary services and should utilize them when appropriate for the benefit of the patient.

## REFERENCES

1. American Psychiatric Association: Diagnostic and Statistical Manual of Mental Disorders, ed. 3. American Psychiatric Association, Washington, D.C., 1980.

2. Harner, R. N.: EEG evaluation of the patient with dementia. In Benson, D. F. and Blumer, D. (eds.): Psychiatric Aspects of Neurologic Disease. Grune and Stratton, New York, 1975, pp. 63–82.

3. Malzberg, B.: Important statistical data about mental illness. In Arieti, S. (ed.): American Handbook of Psychiatry, Vol. 1. Basic Books, New York, 1959, pp. 161–174.

# CHAPTER 2

# History and Behavioral Observations

Most sections of this mental status examination are concerned with the evaluation of specific cognitive functions such as memory and language. But before beginning formal testing, the examiner must take a careful history and make specific and systematic observations of the patient's physical appearance, mood, and behavior.

## HISTORY

The history should be directed toward four primary areas of clinical concern. The first is to establish the presence or absence of classic organic changes (e.g., memory impairment or language disorder). Second, functional psychiatric disorders must also be considered. Although this book is primarily concerned with the changes in emotions and behavior that are seen as a result of organic brain disease, this second area is important for several specific reasons:

1. At times, a specific lesion of the brain (e.g., a tumor of the left frontal lobe) may produce a clinical picture that is indistinguishable from a major functional illness.[19] Cases of depression or mania, schizophrenia, and personality disorders have all been described with organic brain disease. These are classified in the DSM III[1] as organic affective syndrome, organic delusional syndrome, and organic personality syndrome, respectively.
2. It is also common for patients with organic disease to develop associated emotional symptoms such as depression, paranoia, or anxiety.
3. Another important area of overlap between the symptomatology of organic disease and emotional disorders is the problem of pseudodementia, a condition in which the patient has symptoms

and mental status findings that initially suggest a diagnosis of dementia, but eventually prove to be secondary to depression, mania, or other psychiatric disorders.

4. Some patients with a major psychiatric disease (e.g., schizophrenia) will demonstrate cognitive deficits on the mental status examination. This may be due to a concomitant acquired brain lesion or may, in fact, be a part of the total clinical picture of these diseases. When significant cognitive deficits are found in psychiatric patients, the appropriate neurodiagnostic procedures should be conducted.

The third focus of the history must be to establish the patient's premorbid behavior and level of functioning. Information such as education and vocational history are important for establishing expected levels of functioning on the mental status examination. For example, the patient with a third grade education and an inconsistent low-level work history would not be expected to perform at the level of a college graduate engineer or a physician.

The fourth area of importance is the patient's general medical status. Many medical conditions, such as endocrine diseases, chronic renal or hepatic disorders, and chronic alcoholism or drug abuse, adversely affect mental functioning. In some instances, particularly in the elderly, the use of multiple prescription and nonprescription medications can also deleteriously affect mental status.[12] When these conditions do affect mental functioning, they usually produce a confusional state; however, they may mimic a dementia, depression, or other mental disorder. It is important to diagnose such conditions, since they are often reversible with appropriate treatment.

## History Outline

The following elements in the history are particularly important in evaluating a patient with behavior change. Since such patients may not be able to provide a complete and accurate history, it is prudent to obtain the initial information from a family member or other individual who is close to the patient. Even if the patient is able to give a history, corroborative information from a second source is advisable to ensure accuracy.

1. Description of present illness
   a. Nature of onset
   b. Duration of illness
   c. Description of behavioral change associated with illness

2. Other relevant organic behavioral symptoms
    a. Unusual or bizarre behavior (e.g., nocturnal wandering)
    b. Evidence of poor social judgment (e.g., discarding new clothes in the trash or being verbally abusive at social gatherings without provocation); this information should be obtained from someone other than the patient
    c. Attention and concentration problems
    d. Language problems (e.g., word-finding difficulty or tangential verbal responses)
    e. Reading, writing, or calculation difficulty
    f. Memory difficulty
    g. Difficulty with geographic orientation (i.e., getting lost)
3. Psychiatric symptoms
    a. Paranoia
    b. Hallucinations
    c. Delusions
    d. Depression
    e. Anxiety and agitation
4. Past history
    a. Previous neurologic disease or psychiatric problems
    b. Central nervous system infections
    c. Significant head trauma
    d. Seizures
    e. Other medical disease
    f. Drug and alcohol use and misuse
    g. Use of prescription medications and over-the-counter medications
    h. Toxic exposure
5. Birth and developmental history
    a. Brain damage from birth
    b. Developmental delays
        1) Motor
        2) Language
        3) Intellectual
        4) Academic
        5) Emotional and social
6. Educational and vocational history
    a. Highest school grade attained
    b. Adequacy as a student (grade failures)
    c. Vocation
        1) Types of jobs
        2) Frequency of job changes
        3) Recent problems with job

7. Family history
   a. Neurologic or psychiatric disease in another family member
   b. Familial neurologic disease (e.g., Huntington's disease)
   c. Familial predilection for a particular disease process that may involve the central nervous system (e.g., hypertension and stroke)

## BEHAVIORAL OBSERVATION

The primary purpose of this section is to provide a formal framework to assist the examiner in systematically observing behavior. A careful observation of behavior is important because:

1. There are several specific neurobehavioral syndromes (e.g., acute confusional state [delirium], frontal lobe syndrome, and the denial/neglect syndromes) that are diagnosed primarily on the basis of their behavioral manifestations.
2. Such observations provide crucial data to aid in the differential diagnosis between organic and functional disorders.
3. A significant behavioral disturbance may dramatically interfere with subsequent formal testing (e.g., a patient in an organic confusional state will perform poorly on memory testing because of inattention). Sufficient information regarding behavior is not always available from a short period of direct observation and must be obtained from the history provided by family members or other reliable observers.

The discussions of behavior in this chapter are primarily concerned with the identification and description of organic disease and its effects. Extensive discussions of behavior from a psychiatric viewpoint are included in all major psychiatric texts (e.g., Stevenson and Sheppe,[17] Detre and Kupfer,[6] Kaplan and Sadock[10]).

### Physical Appearance

Many patients with either brain disease or functional disorders show characteristic patterns of physical appearance. Classic examples range from that of the patient with organic unilateral neglect with a total lack of attention to dress and care (e.g., shaving and washing) of one side of the body, to that of the obsessive-compulsive neurotic patient who may be scrupulously dressed and groomed and unnecessarily fastidious in matters relating to cleanliness and manner. Obvious neurologic signs, such as hemiplegia or chorea, will not be specifically mentioned. The following aspects of appearance should be noted:

1. General appearance
   a. Descriptive data
      1) Age
      2) Height and weight
   b. General impression of appearance
      1) Appearance for chronologic age
      2) Posture
      3) Facial expression
      4) Eye contact
2. Personal cleanliness
   a. Skin
   b. Hair
   c. Nails
   d. Teeth
   e. Beard
   f. Indications of unilateral neglect
3. Habits of dress
   a. Type of clothing
   b. Cleanliness of clothing
   c. Sloppiness in dressing
   d. Overly fastidious in dress and grooming
   e. Indications of unilateral neglect
4. Motor activity
   a. Level of general activity
      1) Placid versus tense
      2) Hyperkinetic versus hypokinetic
   b. Abnormal posturing
      1) Tics
      2) Facial grimaces
      3) Bizarre gestures
      4) Other involuntary movements

## Mood and General Emotional Status

By mood, we refer to the prevailing and conscious emotional feeling. Emotional status is a general term used to refer to the patient's behavior; it may be evaluated through direct observation of the patient during the examination. Certain organic brain diseases (e.g., frontal lobe disease), as well as psychiatric conditions, may be distinguished by rather characteristic disturbances of mood and emotional status. In addition, any disturbances of mood and emotional status may affect performance on subsequent portions of the mental status examination. Accordingly, a careful and systematic review of the following behavioral components is important. This is not intended to be a complete and definitive psychiatric examination, but rather to provide a framework for the brief assessment of emotional status. This assessment is necessary both for the identification of organically based behavior change and for the initial differentiation of functional and organic disease. Those readers who desire a more comprehensive overview of the psychiatric interpretation of mood and emotional status disturbances may refer to any comprehensive psychiatric text.

1. Mood
   a. Mood normal to the situation
   b. Feeling of sadness (hopelessness, grief, or loss)
   c. Feelings of elation (inappropriate optimism or boastfulness)
   d. Apathy and lack of concern
   e. Constantness or fluctuations in mood
   f. Inappropriate mood: expressed affect is not consistent with the content of thought
2. Emotional status
   a. Degree of cooperation with examiner
   b. Anxiety
   c. Depression
   d. Suspiciousness
   e. Anger
   f. Specific inappropriate emotional responses to particular situations
   g. Reality testing
      1) Delusions (false beliefs)
      2) Illusions (misperceptions of real stimuli)
      3) Hallucinations
      4) Paranoid thinking
   h. Indications of specific neurotic symptoms
      1) Phobias
      2) Chronic anxiety
      3) Obsessive-compulsive thinking and/or behavior
      4) Depression
   i. Abnormalities in language or speech
      1) Neologisms (personal formation of a new word without real meaning except to the patient)
      2) Flight of ideas in thinking and speaking
      3) Loose associations in thinking and speaking

# Clinical Syndromes

There are several distinct clinical entities that are recognized primarily through behavioral observation rather than by specific cognitive testing. These syndromes primarily involve defects in mood and emotional reaction more than alterations in cognition. The diagnosis, therefore, is made by systematic behavioral observation.

## Acute Confusional State (Delirium)

The most common of those behavioral syndromes seen in a general hospital population is the acute confusional state, or delirium. The terms "acute brain syndrome" and "toxic or metabolic encephalopathy" have been employed to describe this state. The acute confusional state has a characteristic constellation of behavioral and historic findings. The onset of symptoms is usually acute (appearing over a period of hours or days).

Generally, the most reliable clinical feature that distinguishes the acute confusional states from other acute organic or functional disorders is a clouding of consciousness. Although this term may seem somewhat vague, it does accurately describe the mental state of the confused patient. Specifically, clouding of consciousness refers both to a dulling of cognitive processes and to a general impairment of alertness.[18] The patients are inattentive and produce incoherent conversations that drift from the central point; they are inconsistent and confabulatory in reporting recent events (e.g., patients may tell the examiner that they have just come back from a walk with a friend when, in fact, they have been in their hospital beds for the entire day); and they often demonstrate fluctuations in their levels of consciousness. Hallucinations, usually visual, and agitation are often present. Some patients who are grossly confusional may be severely agitated and may shout incoherently; these patients usually require restraints to prevent them from disrupting intravenous lines, urinary catheters, and other apparatus. Conversely, other patients may appear superficially normal, but on systematic examination will demonstrate mild degrees of inattention, disorientation, difficulties in carrying out a coherent conversation, and upon specific questioning may admit to nocturnal hallucinations and delusions. The individual patient's confusion is not stable and tends to wax and wane during the day and night. At night, when environmental stimuli are reduced, the confusion and agitation become accentuated.

The confusional state is a very important abnormal behavioral pattern to recognize because it usually represents an acute medical problem rather than a psychiatric condition. Metabolic imbalance, toxic reaction to drugs, sepsis, increased intracranial pressure, or drug withdrawal reactions are the most common causes. Patients in early heart, pulmonary, or hepatic failure may also show confusion. Confusional behavior in the postoperative period is also a common problem. In general, elderly patients, especially those with signs of early dementia, are the most likely to develop confusional states in the above medical situations.

Although psychiatrists are often asked to see these patients because of their abnormal behavior, all such conditions require primary medical treatment. However, even with the administration of proper medical treatment, the confusional state may linger for many days until intracellular balance and general synaptic function are restored. During this period, tranquilizers may be used to calm the patient's agitation.

The confusional state usually results from widespread cortical and subcortical neuronal dysfunction. Cortical dysfunction causes an alteration in the content of consciousness; whereas involvement of the ascending activating system leads to the disturbances of basic arousal. With focal brain disease, confusional behavior may also be seen. This is particularly true in the first few days after an acute cerebrovascular accident or in patients who have brain tumors with associated increased intracranial pressure.

In the patient in a confusional state, further mental status testing will be affected. Inattention plus general cortical dysfunction does not allow the patient to perform adequately on memory, abstract reasoning, or writing tasks.[4] Since the confusion is often slow to clear, definitive mental status testing should be postponed. If the full test is done while the patient is confused, a misdiagnosis of dementia can easily be inadvertently made. Since the changes in the brain are physiologic rather than structural, the patient's level of functioning should eventually return to premorbid levels.

Although the acute onset of inattention, agitation, fluctuating levels of alertness, incoherent speech and train of thought, and visual hallucinations is most often due to a medical condition, the differential diagnosis must include consideration of various functional psychiatric disorders such as acute schizophrenic episode, severe anxiety or panic state, agitated depression, and mania.

The differentiation between the acute organic confusional states and acute severe functional disorders is difficult, but may usually be accurately made with data provided from the patient's medical and psychiatric history, the medical examination, and some aspects of the mental status examination. Alterations in the level of consciousness are almost invariably associated with organic brain disease. Visual hallucinations are more typically seen in organic brain disease; whereas auditory hallucinations are more common in functional psychoses. Systematized delusions are infrequent in the patient in an acute confusional state. In any case where the etiology is unclear, the psychiatrist, neurologist, and primary physician should work closely together to conduct a full evaluation.

## Frontal Lobe Syndrome

Patients with bilateral frontal lobe disease typically do not show dramatic congnitive deficits on formal mental status testing, but they will often demonstrate specific personality changes.[2,20] The most common features of the frontal lobe personality are apathy, both during the examination and toward work and family; euphoria with a tendency toward jocularity; irritability that is short lived; and social inappropriateness.[7] Some patients with frontal lobe disease are predominantly apathetic; they sit and show little interest in any aspect of their environment.[20] In such patients, the apathy is sometimes misconstrued as depression; and lengthy, expensive, and ineffective psychiatric treatment can be undertaken if a careful neurologic examination is not done. Although these patients are primarily apathetic, they may become very irritable and argumentative for short periods of time when sufficiently stressed. Conversely, other patients are primarily loud, jocular, inappropriately intrusive, or socially aggressive. Because of their outgoing behavior, such patients may give the initial impression of interest and productivity. However, this emotional dysinhibition and euphoria does not result in constructive activity. In general, patients with frontal damage have lost both their interest in their environment and their productive social drive. Such patients often fail to maintain job performance, normal family relations, or even personal cleanliness. Since the frontal lobes are the areas of the brain in which reason and emotion interact,[14] bilateral damage may leave the individual with apathy, unchecked emotions, and an intellect without social and emotional guidance.

Behavioral features of the frontal lobe syndrome vary from patient to patient, depending, in part, on the locus of the lesion. Basal-orbital lesions more frequently result in disinhibited, euphoric behavior, with a lack of concern and quick irritability. In contrast, lesions involving the dorsal-lateral convexities tend to produce apathy, reduced drive, depressed mentation, and impaired planning.[19]

The following are two clinical examples of patients with frontal lobe syndromes:

Mrs. L., a 58-year-old housewife, was brought to the hospital by her daughter. The daughter reported that her mother had shown a decreased interest in caring for her house and personal needs for a year.

17

The patient lived alone in a rural area with a few neighbors. The daughter, during an infrequent visit, had noticed a change in her mother's behavior; she showed a lack of interest in conversation, unkempt appearance, a lack of concern about family affairs, and total neglect of personal and household cleanliness. Neighbors had noticed that the patient had discontinued attending church, did very little shopping, and no longer made social visits. Upon examination at hospital admission, Mrs. L. was awake, yet markedly apathetic. She offered no spontaneous conversation and answered all questions with only single-word responses. She had a slow, shuffling gait and had several episodes of incontinence. Neurodiagnostic evaluation (CT scan) demonstrated a large frontal cyst. Surgical exploration with drainage produced a marked behavioral reversal. Within 2 weeks, the patient was walking well, conversing spontaneously, and was no longer apathetic or incontinent. Mrs. L. represented the primarily apathetic variation of the frontal lobe syndrome.

The following is a case that demonstrates the dysinhibition, social inappropriateness, and jocularity that may be associated with the underlying apathy in some cases of this syndrome. Mr. N. was 65 years old when brought to the hospital by his wife. Her chief complaint was that her husband's mind was deranged. The wife stated that her husband had always been a great joker but had used proper social restraint until about 4 or 5 years ago. At that time, he began to show excessive candor in his remarks to friends and acquaintances. His usual outgoing personality gave way to flippancy and arrogance. His prior restraint was decreased, and he approached each social situation with an almost aggressive egotism, with much showing off and boasting.

Over the past years, he had lost regard for his personal cleanliness, bathing and shaving only at his wife's behest. His wife also reported that his memory had started to fail and that he confabulated on occasion. At one point, she had bought a new lawn mower and brought it home with the handle disassembled. She had asked him to put the handle together and to put it on the mower; he had been totally unable to do so.

Later in his course, he became quite agitated and paranoid. He wandered around the neighborhood and often told strangers fantastic tales, the last being that he was an undercover agent for the FBI. His judgment in other matters also deteriorated. The last time he drove the car, he went through a stop sign and joked about it with his wife. These last events prompted his referral to the hospital.

Examination revealed an inattentive, restless, socially inappropriate man who was physically unkempt, with uncombed hair, uncut fingernails and toenails, and messy clothes. He exhibited some paranoia, asking if his medicine (Thorazine) was some sort of poison; several times during the examination, he attempted to leave the room and was obviously agitated. His thought processes were extremely concrete, and he performed poorly on virtually all aspects of the mental status examination. During the hospital period, he became quite upset and irritable, especially at night, and was somewhat aggressive with several nurses. The CT scan revealed frontotemporal atrophy with greatly enlarged frontal horns and widened sulci. The presumptive diagnosis in this case was Pick's disease. He died in 1982, and the autopsy verified that diagnosis.

If the behavioral manifestations of the frontal lobe syndrome are present, the following neurologic diseases should be considered in the differential diagnosis: (1) tumors—subfrontal meningiomas, pituitary adenomas, or primary brain tumors; (2) head trauma with frontal contusions; (3) Pick's disease; (4) general paresis; (5) communicating hydrocephalus; and (6) Huntington's disease. Any patient with extensive cortical disease (e.g., late Alzheimer's disease, multiple cortical infarcts, or traumatic or postinfectious encephalopathy) will show some of the behavior changes seen in the patient with frontal lobe disease. However, such patients also show evidence of severe cognitive dysfunction and other indications of involvement of other brain areas.

Disease of the frontal lobes may be difficult to evaluate clinically because of the relative absence of clear-cut cognitive changes with lesions of this area.[2,21] There are, however, some clinical tests that can be used to assess frontal lobe functioning. These are primarily alternating sequencing tasks and have been shown by Luria[13] to be impaired in cases with extensive frontal lobe disease.

Alternating Sequences—Visual Pattern Completion. *Directions.* Present the patient with the following visual patterns on individual sheets of white paper (Fig. 2-1). Tell the patient to reproduce the stimulus figure and then to continue the alternating sequence. If necessary, give additional elaboration of the directions to ensure that the patient understands the nature of the test. Do not correct the errors or provide additional cues after the patient begins the task.

*Scoring.* Patients with intact motor and sensory systems should be capable of completing these sequences without error. A loss of the sequence or perseveration in the reproduction of sequences is suggestive of a loss of the ability to move from one motor movement to another and an inability to shift sets efficiently. Examples of common errors are shown in Figure 2-2.

Alternating Motor Patterns. *Directions.* This test consists of a series of changes in hand position. They have been adapted from Luria[13] and are described in greater detail in that source.

1. Fist-Palm-Side Test

Tell the patient to repeatedly hit the top of the desk, first with a fist, then with an open palm, and then with the side of the hand. Demon-

FIGURE 2-1. Test items for Visual Pattern Completion Test.

strate the task once, and then tell the patient to perform the task until told to stop. Performance for 15 to 20 seconds should suffice to assess the adequacy of these alternating movements.

### 2. Fist-Ring Test

Instruct the patient to extend his or her arm several times, first with the hand in a fist, and then with the thumb and forefinger opposed to form a ring. Demonstrate the action, and then tell the patient to perform the action. With successive extensions of the arm, the patient alternates between these two positions.

### 3. Reciprocal Coordination Test

This is an alternation test that utilizes both hands. Initially, the patient places both hands on the desk, one in a fist and one with the fingers extended palm down. Tell the patient to rapidly alternate the position of the two hands (simultaneously extending the fingers of one hand while making a fist with the other). Demonstrate the nature of the task.

FIGURE 2-2. Common errors in Visual Pattern Completion Test.

*Scoring.* Normal patients should have no difficulty in easily mastering these alternating sequences after one or two attempts.[13] Accordingly, any appreciable disruption of the smooth performance of these tasks is indicative of dysfunction of the premotor areas of the cerebral cortex.

Denial and Neglect

In some patients, a brain lesion may produce a striking degree of denial of illness. The following recent case is an excellent example:

A surgeon was finishing an operation when his assistant noticed that the surgeon's left arm had suddenly become weak and his speech slurred. The surgeon was immediately put on a stretcher and was brought to the intensive care unit, where one of us saw him within minutes. The patient's arm and face were still weak, but when asked, he replied that "it is OK." His weakness was specifically pointed out to him, and his comment was, "I really don't recognize any weakness."

This degree of denial does not seem to be the result of a strengthening of the psychologic defense mechanisms but is a more basic and unusual organic behavior change. Clinically, there is a spectrum of denial and neglect syndromes, which ranges from explicit denial of illness (e.g., the example above) as the most severe behavioral abnormality, to a mild inability to recognize stimulation on one side of the body during bilateral simultaneous stimulation (inattention or extinction). The patient with gross denial may deny total cortical blindness (Anton's syndrome) or a severe hemiparesis (anosognosia).

In many patients with denial, the denial is more implicit than explicit. For example, when asked about the illness, the patient may not actively deny that he or she is ill, but may say that the hospitalization is for tests to evaluate mild joint pain or some similar benign condition. Some patients state that they are not really in a hospital at all, but merely in a rest facility or hotel (reduplication of place or paramnesia). Such patients will often make elaborate excuses of fatigue when asked to perform with the paralyzed limb (confabulation) and on occasion will even claim that the weak arm is not theirs at all (reduplication of body parts). The surgeon mentioned above, for instance, claimed, on the following day, that he "had some arthritis" in his left arm and that was the reason for his not moving it.

Hemiplegic patients who deny weakness are a great problem in rehabilitation because they are unaware of their weakness and tend to fall repeatedly. Our patient tried to walk to the bathroom on the first day after his right hemisphere stroke and fell, fracturing his left clavicle.

Some patients do not demonstrate frank denial but do have a dramatic neglect of one side of the body. Such patients may shave only one side of the face, use only one sleeve of their robe, and fail to use one side of the body even though paralysis is not present. These patients also neglect one half of the extrapersonal environment, even in the absence of a visual field defect. For example, patients may fail to respond to a visitor who approaches them from their involved side. Patients may also show neglect on drawing tasks. Examples of this type of neglect are shown in Figure 2-3.

The most subtle form of neglect is an inattention to one side of the body when both sides are simultaneously stimulated. This tendency to suppress or to extinguish the stimuli on the involved side is discussed in detail in Chapter 4.

The lesion that most frequently causes the denial and neglect syndromes is a nondominant-hemisphere lesion, most frequently vascular in etiology.[5] A specific lesion locus within the right hemisphere has not yet been established. Subcortical as well as cortical structures may be involved. Gross explicit denial is an uncommon behavioral finding that is most frequently seen during the acute stages of a vascular accident and is frequently associated with a degree of confusion. Unilateral neglect may be seen as a chronic effect of parietal lesions, predominantly in the nondominant hemisphere. The actual neuropsychologic and neurophysiologic mechanisms underlying these syndromes are not completely understood. Patients with frontal lobe disease may also show evidence of denial. For a review of this problem, see Heilman and associates,[8] Weinstein and Friedland,[22] and Weinstein and Kahn.[23]

Apathy vs. Depression

Apathy, lack of interest in the environment, and psychomotor slowing (psychomotor retardation) are frequently observed in patients with psychiatric depressive illness. Essentially identical symptoms, however, are characteristic of a variety of organic brain diseases as well: in particular, dementia, frontal lobe lesions, and right-hemisphere lesions. Many inexperienced clinicians have an unfortunate tendency to equate apathy with depression. Apathy is but a single symptom and, in isolation, never justifies the diagnosis of depression. The importance of differentiating apathy of organic etiology from functional depression cannot be overstressed.

Depression is a specific affective disorder that is a syndrome composed of many symptoms. The accepted criteria for establishing a diagnosis of a major depressive disorder are as follows:

A. Dysphoric mood (sadness, hopelessness, and irritability) or loss of interest in all or almost all usual activities

FIGURE 2-3. Examples of neglect on drawing test.

B. Four of the following, persistent for at least 2 weeks:
  1. Poor appetite
  2. Insomnia or hypersomnia
  3. Psychomotor agitation or retardation
  4. Loss of interest
  5. Loss of energy
  6. Feelings of worthlessness
  7. Complaints of decreased concentration and thinking ability
  8. Recurrent thoughts of death or suicide

Any patient presenting with apathy of nonacute onset as an initial symptom should be carefully screened for the possible presence of a primary depressive disorder before the physician entertains a diagnosis of organic disease.

One of the most common diagnostic dilemmas is the differentiation between depression and early dementia. Both conditions are relatively common in the older population, and more importantly, they share many common features. Because of these similarities, a misdiagnosis of one for the other is all too easily made. The significance of such an error is obvious. To tell a depressed individual that he or she is demented is a devastating error, but no less significant than overlooking a frontal meningioma while treating the patient for depression.

One can easily see why diagnostic confusion may occur; both conditions can present with complaints of apathy, loss of interest in work and pleasurable activities, preoccupation with minor or imagined physical complaints, difficulty concentrating, memory loss, and a general inability to keep up with the demands of everyday life. The problem is further compounded in the elderly; these patients, when depressed, do not manifest depressive mood as dramatically as do younger patients. The elderly depressive patient also demonstrates fewer crying spells, less expressed sadness, less suicidal ideation (though there is no less threat of actual suicide), less expressed guilt, and less self-deprecation.[9] The elderly depressive patient may also show subtle cognitive deficits on formal mental status testing. No specific pattern of deficits is seen, and the deficits are usually mild.[3] Mild problems with concentration, memory, and arithmetic are common. There may be a paucity of details on drawings and, in general, impaired performance on any task that requires the marshaling of significant mental energy.

Because of the similarity of clinical presentation, it is not surprising that many elderly depressive patients are initially diagnosed as having a dementia.[15] The term pseudodementia has been applied to those patients in whom the initial diagnostic impression is of a dementia, yet on careful evaluation and follow-up, the patients' symptoms prove to be secondary to depression or another emotional disorder.[11,16]

The differentiation of true early dementia from pseudodementia is not always easy. Wells[24] has tabulated the major features that he feels can help make this distinction; these are summarized below.

| | Pseudodementia | Dementia |
|---|---|---|
| A. Clinical course and history | 1. onset fairly well demarcated | 1. onset indistinct |
| | 2. history short | 2. history quite long before consultation |
| | 3. rapidly progressive | 3. early deficits often go unnoticed |
| | 4. history of previous psychiatric difficulty or recent life crisis | 4. previous psychiatric problems or emotional crisis uncommon |
| B. Clinical behavior | 1. detailed, elaborate complaints of cognitive dysfunction | 1. little complaint of cognitive loss |
| | 2. put out little effort on examination items | 2. struggle with cognitive tasks |
| | 3. affective change often present | 3. usually apathetic with shallow emotions |
| | 4. behavior does not reflect cognitive loss | 4. behavior compatible with cognitive loss |
| | 5. rarely has exacerbation at night | 5. nocturnal accentuation of dysfunction common |
| C. Examination findings | 1. frequently answers "I don't know" before even trying | 1. usually will try on items |
| | 2. inconsistent memory loss for both recent and remote items | 2. memory loss for recent events worse than remote |
| | 3. may have particular memory gaps | 3. no specific memory gaps |
| | 4. in general, performance is inconsistent | 4. rather consistently impaired performance |

In our experience, if the examiner takes his or her time and encourages optimum performance from the patient, the pseudodementia patient will show good performance that is far better than would be expected from the nature and severity of the complaints.

The problem of pseudodementia is most commonly seen in the elderly depressed patient; however, hysterical conversion reactions, mania, and high levels of anxiety can all produce a picture of dementia on mental status examination. In these cases, it is the inattention and racing thoughts that preclude adequate performance on the examination. It is rewarding to see a patient with "pseudodementia" because, with appropriate treatment, the patient's mental status will revert to normal, premorbid levels.

# SUMMARY

Organic brain lesions may cause a multiplicity of behavioral syndromes, some of which are characteristic of specific clinical conditions. The examiner must be prepared to make a systematic evaluation of the patient's behavior and be able to recognize the major neurobehavioral syndromes.

# REFERENCES

1. American Psychiatric Association: Diagnostic and Statistical Manual of Mental Disorders (DSM III). American Psychiatric Association, Washington, D.C., 1980.
2. Black, F. W.: Cognitive deficits in patients with unilateral war-related frontal lobe lesions. J Clin Psychol 32:307, 1976.
3. Caine, E. D.: Pseudodementia: Current concepts and future directions. Arch Gen Psychiatry 38:1359, 1981.
4. Chédru, F. and Geschwind, N.: Writing disturbances in acute confusional states. Neuropsychologia 10:343, 1972.
5. Critchley, M.: The Parietal Lobes. Edward Arnold & Co, London, 1953.
6. Detre, T. P. and Kupfer, D. F.: Psychiatric history and mental status examination. In Freedman, A., Kaplan, H., and Sadock, B. (eds.): Comprehensive Textbook of Psychiatry, Vol. 1. Williams & Wilkins, Baltimore, 1975, pp. 724–735.
7. Hécaen, H. and Albert, M. L.: Disorders of mental functioning related to frontal lobe pathology. In Benson, D. F. and Blumer, D. (eds.): Psychiatric Aspects of Neurologic Disease. Grune & Stratton, New York, 1975, pp. 137–149.
8. Heilman, K. M., et al: Localization of lesions in neglect. In Kertesz, A. (ed.): Localization in Neuropsychology. Academic Press, New York, 1983, pp. 471–492.
9. Janowsky, D. S.: Pseudodementia in the elderly: Differential diagnosis and treatment. J Clin Psychiatry 43:19, 1982.
10. Kaplan, H. I. and Sadock, B. J.: Modern Synopsis of Comprehensive Textbook of Psychiatry. Williams & Wilkins, Baltimore, 1981.
11. Kiloh, L. G.: Pseudo-dementia. Acta Psychiatr Scand 37:336, 1961.
12. Levenson, A. J. (ed.): Neuropsychiatric Side-effects of Drugs in the Elderly. Raven Press, New York, 1979.
13. Luria, A. R.: Traumatic Aphasia. Moulton and Co, The Hague, 1970.
14. Nauta, W. J. H.: The problem of the frontal lobe: A reinterpretation. J Psychiatr Res 8:167, 1971.
15. Nott, P. N. and Fleminger, J. J.: Presenile dementia: The difficulties of early diagnosis. Acta Psychiatr Scand 51:210, 1975.
16. Post, F.: Dementia, depression and pseudo-dementia. In Benson, D. F. and Blumer, D. (eds.): Psychiatric Aspects of Neurologic Disease. Grune & Stratton, New York, 1975, pp. 99–120.
17. Stevenson, I. and Sheppe, W. M.: The psychiatric examination. In Arieti, S. (ed.): American Handbook of Pyschiatry, Vol. 1. Basic Books, New York, 1974, pp. 1156–1186.
18. Strub, R. L.: Acute confusional state. In Benson, D. F. and Blumer, D. (eds.): Psychiatric Aspects of Neurologic Disease, Vol. II. Grune & Stratton, New York, 1982, pp. 1–21.

19. Stuss, D. T. and Benson, D. F.: Frontal lobe lesions and behavior. In Kertesz, A. (ed.): Localization in Neuropsychology. Academic Press, New York, 1983, pp. 429–454.
20. Stuss, D. T. and Benson, D. F.: Neuropsychological studies of the frontal lobes. Psychol Bull 95:3, 1984.
21. Teuber, H. L.: The riddle of frontal lobe function in man. In Warren, J. and Alert, K. (eds.): The Frontal Granular Cortex and Behavior. McGraw-Hill, New York, 1964, pp. 410–440.
22. Weinstein, E. A. and Friedland, R. P.: Hemi-Inattention and Hemispheric Specialization. Advances in Neurology, Vol. 18. Raven Press, New York, 1977.
23. Weinstein, E. A. and Kahn, R. L.: Denial of Illness. Charles C. Thomas, Springfield, Ill, 1955.
24. Wells, C. E.: Pseudodementia. Am J Psychiatry 136:895, 1979.

CHAPTER 3

# Levels of Consciousness

The initial step in administering a formal mental status examination is the determination of the patient's level of consciousness. This basic brain function determines the patient's ability to relate both to self and to environment. Any disturbance of this elementary function will almost invariably affect the higher-level mental processes that constitute the major portion of the examination. The term consciousness is multifaceted; in testing, it is important to distinguish between the content of consciousness and basic arousal.[7] Content refers to higher cognitive and emotional functioning; whereas arousal refers to the activation of the cortex from the ascending activating system (brain stem reticular formation and the diffuse thalamic projection system). Both content and arousal can vary independently, and the final level of consciousness represents a dynamic balance between cortical and ascending activating systems. This chapter deals with the clinical aspects of basic arousal; a discussion of changes in the content of consciousness is included in subsequent sections of the book.

## TERMINOLOGY AND EVALUATION

There are many general terms used to describe the basic levels or states of consciousness. These levels represent points on a continuum from full alertness to deep coma. Most clinicians distinguish five principal levels: (1) alertness, (2) lethargy or somnolence, (3) obtundation, (4) stupor or semicoma, and (5) coma. Alertness implies that the patient is awake and fully aware of normal external and internal stimuli. Barring paralysis, the patient can respond normally to any normal stimulus. The alert patient is able to interact in a meaningful way with the examiner. In cases of total paralysis, eye contact or eye movement may be adequate to establish this interaction. Because there are unusual coma-like states in which alertness is simulated, we feel that an observation of alertness should be predicated upon the clinician's impression that meaningful interpersonal interaction is taking place. Alertness, per se, does not imply the inherent capacity to focus attention, a topic to be discussed in detail in Chapter 4.

Lethargy is a state in which the patient is not fully alert and tends to drift off to sleep when not stimulated. In such patients, spontaneous movements are decreased and awareness is limited. When aroused, these patients usually cannot pay close attention to the examiner. The lethargic patient often loses the train of thought and wanders from topic to topic in conversation. It is difficult to assess memory, calculations, and abstract thinking in these patients because of their inattention and wandering thought processes. If a full mental status examination is performed in a lethargic patient, the results must be interpreted with caution.

Obtundation is a term used by many physicians to refer to a transitional state between lethargy and stupor. The obtunded patient is difficult to arouse and, when aroused, is confusional. Usually, constant stimulation is required to elicit even marginal cooperation from the patient. Meaningful mental status testing is usually futile. The obtunded patient is, by our definition, in an acute confusional state or quiet delirium.

The terms stupor and semicoma are used to describe patients who respond only to persistent and vigorous stimulation. The stuporous patient does not rouse spontaneously and, when aroused by the examiner, is able only to groan or mumble and move restlessly in the bed. In such a patient, there is extensive brain dysfunction; thus, no meaningful assessment of the content of mental functioning is possible.

Coma is a term traditionally applied to those patients who are completely unarousable. In coma, the patient will neither respond to any external stimulation nor respond spontaneously to an internal stimulus. If coma is thus defined as a state in which no evidence of behavioral response to stimulation is present, the term can serve as an absolute end point on the scale of consciousness or arousability. Some clinicians make a distinction between light coma and deep coma. In light coma, the patient may demonstrate reflex (e.g., decorticate or decerebrate) movements but no meaningful or purposeful movements; whereas in deep coma, no motor response is seen. Stupor and coma will not be further discussed here; the interested reader is referred to Plum and Posner[7] and Fisher[2] for extensive discussions of these states.

Each of the above mentioned terms is qualitative in nature and encompasses a wide range of possible points on the continuum of consciousness. Such terms lack the objectivity and reliability that can be achieved with a more objective assessment scheme. We suggest amending any qualitative term such as "lethargy" with a series of short statements that describe the level of stimulus necessary to arouse the patient and the actual behavioral response. First, indicate the intensity of stimulation needed to arouse the patient: (1) calling the patient's name in a normal conversational tone, (2) calling in a loud voice, (3) light touch on the arm, (4) vigorous shaking of the patient's shoulder, or (5) painful stimulation. Second, describe the patient's highest level responses: (1) degree and quality of movement, (2) presence and coherence of speech, or (3) presence of eye opening and eye contact with the examiner. Finally, describe what the patient does upon cessation of stimulation.

This information can be recorded in a single statement. As examples: (1) Patient lethargic: name called in a normal tone of voice; patient opened eyes, pulled self part way up in bed, mumbled "Why ya bothering me," then closed eyes and went back to sleep. (2) Patient obtunded: responds to loud shouting with restless movements of all extremities and brief eye opening; speech is mumbled and incoherent; when stimulation discontinued, patient returns to sleep. (3) Patient stuporous: does not respond to voice, but will respond to vigorous shaking of shoulder accompanied by loud calling of patient's name; patient responds with a groan and aimless movement of left extremities; eyes remain closed.

These types of descriptions provide much more data on the patient's arousability and capacity for interaction than the simple terms "lethargy," "obtundation," or "stupor." It is helpful to make a chart in the progress notes so that a rapid assessment of changing levels of consciousness can be made. Table 3-1 is an example of a patient with head trauma who had a subdural hematoma. As shifts of nurses and doctors change, subtle changes in the patient's condition are easily appreciated by comparing the notes of previous observers. This system is applicable to any patient whose illness causes a decrease in the level of awareness.

Teasdale and Jennett[4,9] have demonstrated the practicality of this type of reporting system for patients with head injury. They have developed what has become known as The Glasgow Coma, or Responsiveness, Scale. It follows the same conceptual scheme that we have used but has the advantage of providing a numerical score to denote the actual level of consciousness. Each level of response in the three response categories (i.e., eye opening, verbal, motor) is given a numerical value. The response is the patient's best response; it does not, however, take into account the level of stimulus required for its elicitation. The scale items and the quantitative ratings for specific responses are presented in Table 3-2.

The level of responsiveness can be assessed objectively at regular intervals and plotted in graphic form. The time scale can be hourly, daily, or any selected interval. Table 3-3 is an example of such use of the scale.

TABLE 3-1. Patient's Responses to Stimulation

| | Level of Consciousness | Stimulus Necessary to Rouse Patient | Movement | Vocalization | Eye Opening | Comments |
|---|---|---|---|---|---|---|
| 8 PM | Lethargy | Loud voice | Moved all limbs; got up on elbow | Mumbled something about being tired | Yes, with eye contact | Odor of alcohol on breath |
| 12 AM | Lethargy | Loud voice plus gentle shaking | Moved all limbs; no attempt to rise | Incoherent mumbling | Yes, but no sustained eye contact | Questionable Babinski sign |
| 4 AM | Stupor | Loud voice plus vigorous shaking | Slight movement of all extremities, but right arm not moving well | Groans | Attempted to open eyes to command | Left pupil larger than right, not as reactive; now positive Babinski on right |

Table 3-2. Glasgow Coma Scale*

| Category of Response | Response | Points |
|---|---|---|
| Eye Opening | Spontaneous | 4 |
| | To speech | 3 |
| | To pain | 2 |
| | Nil | 1 |
| Best Verbal Response | Oriented | 5 |
| | Confused conversation | 4 |
| | Inappropriate words | 3 |
| | Incomprehensible | 2 |
| | Nil | 1 |
| Best Motor Response | Obeys | 6 |
| | Localizes | 5 |
| | Withdraws | 4 |
| | Abnormal flexion (decorticate) | 3 |
| | Extends (decerebrate) | 2 |
| | Nil | 1 |

*Adapted from Jennett and Teasdale,[4] p. 78.

# ANATOMY AND CLINICAL IMPLICATIONS

The basic brain structure that is responsible for arousal is the ascending activating system. This system originates in the brain stem reticular formation and extends to the cortex via the diffuse or nonspecific thalamic projection system.[6]

There is a group of specialized reticular neurons in the tegmental portion of the midbrain and upper pons that has the specific capacity to activate higher centers. These cells are located in a perimedian portion in the brain stem and receive collateral input from most ascending and descending fiber systems. Stimulation to the skin of the hand, for example, will send information to the activating system as well as the sensory nuclei in the thalamus. Reticular stimulation alerts widespread areas of the cortex and subcortex to the fact that an external stimulus is being applied. By this mechanism, the activating system maintains a constant, albeit fluctuating, stimulation of the higher centers. Without this steady input, the cortex cannot function efficiently; thus, the patient cannot think clearly, learn effectively, or relate meaningfully. Any damage or suppression of this system renders the patient difficult to arouse and inefficient in performance. Specific lesions such as infarcts or hemorrhages of the reticular formation lead to total disruption of arousal and, thus, to coma. Pressure on the midbrain from hippocampal or uncal herniation will cause a change in the level of consciousness, which starts

TABLE 3-3. Glasgow Coma Scale Graph

| Patient's | Response | Date | 12 PM | 2 PM | 4 PM | 6 PM | 8 PM | 10 PM | 12 AM |
|---|---|---|---|---|---|---|---|---|---|
| Eye Opening | Spontaneous | | | | | | | | |
| | To Speech | | | | | | | | |
| | To Pain | | | | | | | | |
| | None | | | | | | | | |
| Best Verbal Response | Oriented | | | | | | | | |
| | Confused | | | | | | | | |
| | Inappropriate | | | | | | | | |
| | Incomprehensible | | | | | | | | |
| | None | | | | | | | | |
| Best Motor Response | Obeying | | | | | | | | |
| | Localizing | | | | | | | | |
| | Withdraws | | | | | | | | |
| | Flexing | | | | | | | | |
| | Extending | | | | | | | | |
| | None | | | | | | | | |
| | Coma Score | | 12 | 11 | 8 | 6 | 6 | 4 | |

34

as lethargy but may progress to coma. Drug intoxication, disturbances in metabolic balance, and sepsis cause alterations in both reticular and cortical functioning. This leads to alterations not only in arousal, but also in the content of consciousness.

If there is damage to the extension of the brain stem reticular system in the thalamus or hypothalamus, the full picture of coma will not result. Such lesions disconnect the reticulocortical pathways and cause the patients to display various interesting alterations in arousal. Since the brain stem portion of the system is intact, reticular activity innervates the nuclei of the extraocular nerves, and the patients can open their eyes and look about. The cortex, however, is not sufficiently stimulated to produce voluntary movement or speech. These patients are in a coma-like state.

These unusual coma-like states are interesting because of the nature and degree of disturbed awareness. Some authors combine all such cases under the rubrics of akinetic mutism or persistent vegetative states, while others prefer to separate the patients into many subcategories. Regardless of the terminology employed, the pathology and clinical appearance of each subcategory is relatively distinct and can usually be recognized by a thorough examiner. The primary feature of these disorders is the patient's uncanny appearance of awareness. Such patients lie in bed with their eyes open and look about the room. Eye contact with others is variable. Sometimes eye movements seem random; but on other occasions, real interpersonal eye contact appears to take place. Other than this somewhat unnerving visual scanning, the patients remain relatively immobile and mute. It is the dichotomy between this apparent visual alertness and the lack of speech and movement that differentiates this group of patients from those in stupor or coma.

Regardless of their superficial similarity, each subgroup has its own distinct features, and it is often possible to clinically differentiate the various states. The term akinetic mutism seems best reserved for cases in which damage is restricted to either the midbrain/subthalamic region or to the septal region. The midbrain lesion causes a syndrome that is described as an apathetic akinetic mutism. These patients are difficult to arouse; but once aroused, they can move all extremities, mutter a few intelligible words, and look directly at the examiner for a few moments. They then turn away or drift back into sleep. Subtle muscle stretch reflex changes, possible extensor toe signs, extraocular muscle involvement, and pupillary abnormalities may be seen. This condition was originally described in a patient with a third ventricular cyst,[1] but the most common cause is occlusion of the small vessels entering the brain stem from the tip of the basilar artery.[8] This lesion interrupts the ascending activating system but not the corticospinal and corticobulbar tracts.

Accordingly, the patients are able to open their eyes and make some movement and sound, but they are not able to respond fully.

Patients with lesions that involve the septal area, anterior hypothalamus, cingulate gyri, or bilateral orbital frontal cortex are also akinetic and mute, but they appear much more alert. They are awake most of the day and insomniac at night; their eyes remain open when awake. These patients often have violent behavioral outbursts during arousal (septal rage). Coma vigil is a term that has been used to describe such patients. This syndrome is seen with rupture of anterior communicating artery aneurysms, deep frontal lobe tumors, and anterior cingulate gyrus tumors. These patients may have increased reflexes in the legs with Babinski signs from corticospinal tract involvement, difficulty with temperature control from anterior hypothalamic damage, and primitive reflexes (snout and grasp) from mesial frontal lobe damage. They do not have pupillary or extraocular muscle paresis. These neurologic signs plus the more apparent alertness of these patients will frequently differentiate them clinically from apathetic akinetic mute patients.

Patients with diffuse damage to the cortical mantle from anoxia, hypoglycemia, or circulatory or metabolic embarrassment will frequently survive in a state clinically similar to coma vigil. Their eyes are open and randomly survey the room. Brain stem reflexes are intact, but there is bilateral decortication with double hemiplegia and primitive reflexes. This condition has been termed the apallic state[5] because of the diffuse damage to the neocortex, or neopallium. Because of the dramatic neurologic deficit, this state should be easily distinguished from the akinetic mute states.

The term persistent vegetative state has been used to describe patients surviving severe head injury who are clinically similar to patients in the apallic state.[3] The brain lesions are widespread at both the cortical and subcortical levels, and neurologic findings differ in each case depending upon the specific loci of the lesions. Since the term apallic state has never gained widespread acceptance, persistent vegetative state is often used for any patient with widespread brain disease and no ability to meaningfully interact with the environment.

The locked-in syndrome[7] must also be recognized and differentiated from the above states. In this condition, there is a lesion (hemorrhage or infarct) in the upper pontine tegmentum that interrupts all corticospinal and corticobulbar fibers at the level of the abducens and facial nuclei. Clinically, patients are unable to speak, swallow, smile, or move their limbs. In some cases, lateral gaze is also paralyzed. The entire central nervous system above the level of the lesion is intact, and the patient is literally disconnected from his motor system. The patient is "locked-in" and is able to communicate with onlookers only by eye movements.

Table 3-4 is a composite of the clinical features of each of these coma-like states. These features plus the clinical history should enable the examiner to differentiate most of these complicated cases.

A final condition that deserves mention in this section is the state of psychogenic unresponsiveness (hysteric coma-like state). This condition constitutes 1 percent of all patients presenting to a medical emergency room in an unresponsive state.[7] Careful examination reveals normal respiration, heart rate, and blood pressure. Muscle tone is usually decreased, but there is frequently inconsistent limb tone. All bulbar reflexes (doll's phenomenon, caloric stimulation, gag, corneal, and pupil) are intact. Muscle stretch reflexes are symmetrical, and neurologic examination strongly suggests that the condition is psychogenic. Frequently, the patient will make inconsistent responses, such as blinking on corneal testing before the cornea is touched. Any inconsistent response gives the examiner additional confidence that he or she is not dealing with an organic coma. Do not diagnose psychogenic unresponsiveness too hastily; the misdiagnosis of a true coma as hysteria is far more serious than the reverse.

All of the conditions discussed above represent disturbances of arousal caused by brain lesions or psychiatric illness. Not all alterations in levels of alertness are pathologic, however. Sleep, for instance, is a natural fluctuation in the level of consciousness. Any degree of fatigue or sleepiness can adversely affect performance on mental status testing even though an organic lesion is not present. Patients with brain disease will continue to have an underlying diurnal sleep/wake cycle that is superimposed upon any organic decrease in alertness. It may be difficult to determine the relative effects of sleep and pathologic alterations in the level of consciousness, but the examiner must consider both factors in the evaluation. For example, the patient with head trauma who is difficult to arouse on morning rounds may only be asleep and not suffering from increasing intracranial pressure. In these critical cases, the observed level of awareness is not the only clinical factor that determines the necessity for therapeutic intervention. The patient's neurologic status and overall hospital course must also be considered.

## SUMMARY

Consciousness is the most rudimentary of all mental functions, and its level must be determined first in any mental status examination. Any alteration in the level of consciousness will decrease the efficiency of cortical functioning, and thereby significantly decrease the validity of the subsequent steps in the mental status examination. In the patient

TABLE 3-4. Diagnostic Features of Coma-like States

| Diagnosis | Level of Consciousness | Voluntary Movement | Speech | Eye Responses | Limb Tone | Reflexes |
|---|---|---|---|---|---|---|
| Akinetic mute (apathetic—midbrain) | Lethargy. | Little and infrequent; but when sufficiently stimulated, can move *all* extremities purposefully. | With stimulation, can produce normal, short phrases. | Open when stimulated. Usually good eye contact. | Usually normal; sometimes slight increase. | Can be normal. Occasionally asymmetrical with pathologic reflexes. |
| Akinetic mute (coma—vigil—septal) | Wakeful, with occasional outbursts. Some patients are somnolent. | Little but purposeful; arms usually move much better than legs. | Little; can occasionally produce normal phrases. Also, can have outbursts of unintelligible utterances. | Open during much of the day in most patients. Eye contact variable. | Often increased in legs. | Frequently have increased leg reflexes. Babinski signs, snout, grasp often present. |
| Apallic state (decorticate) | Awake; no meaningful interaction with environment. | No or little purposeful movement; mostly reflex or mass movements. | None or occasional grunting. | Open, searching, but no real eye contact. | Increased in all extremities. Extremities often in flexion. | Increased in all extremities with pathologic reflexes. |
| Persistent vegetative state | Awake; no or little interaction with environment. | Usually little or none, depending upon areas of brain damaged. Mostly primitive postural reflexes. | None or occasional grunts or groans. Some patients produce a few words. | Open, searching, but no real eye contact. | Variable, usually increased. Extremities often in flexion. | Variable, usually increased with pathologic reflexes. |
| Locked-in syndrome | Awake and alert; able to communicate meaningfully with examiners by eye movement. | None or slight, except for eye movement. | None. | Open, with normal following and good eye contact. Some patients have restricted lateral gaze. | Increased. | Increased in all extremities. |

with diminished alertness, only the more obvious changes in higher cognitive function can be validly documented.

The arousal aspect of consciousness is controlled by the ascending activating system. Any damage to or dysfunction of this subcortical system alters alertness and thus, secondarily, affects cortical activity.

## REFERENCES

1. Cairns, H., et al: Akinetic mutism with an epidermoid cyst of the third ventricle. Brain 64:273, 1941.
2. Fisher, C. M.: The neurological examination of the comatose patient. Acta Neurol Scand (Suppl.) 36:1, 1969.
3. Jennett, B. and Plum, F.: Persistent vegetative state after brain damage. Lancet 1:734, 1972.
4. Jennett, B. and Teasdale, G.: Assessment of impaired consciousness. In Jennett, B. and Teasdale, G.: Management of Head Injuries. FA Davis, Philadelphia, 1981, pp. 77-93.
5. Kretschmer, E.: Das Appalische Syndrom. Z Gesamte Neurol Psychiat 169:576, 1940.
6. Magoun, H.: The Waking Brain. Charles C Thomas, Springfield, Ill, 1963.
7. Plum, F. and Posner, J.: Diagnosis of Stupor and Coma. FA Davis, Philadelphia, 1980.
8. Segarra, J. and Angelo, J.: Anatomical determinants of behavior change. In Benton, A. (ed.): Behavioral Change in Cerebral Vascular Disease. Harper & Row, New York, 1970, pp. 3-14.
9. Teasdale, G. and Jennett, B.: Assessment of coma and impaired consciousness. Lancet 2:81, 1974.

# CHAPTER 4

# Attention

After determining the level of consciousness, a careful assessment of attention is the next step in the formal mental status examination. The patient's ability to sustain attention over time must be established before the more complex functions such as memory, language, and abstract thinking are evaluated. It is of no value to ask the patient to remember the details of a story if he is repeatedly distracted by the nurse passing in the hall, a noise in the next room, or cars in the street. When a patient is inattentive and distractible, he or she is unable to assimilate the information to be tested.

Attention refers to the patient's ability to attend to a specific stimulus without being distracted by extraneous environmental stimuli. This capacity for focusing on a single stimulus is in contrast to the concept of alertness. Alertness is a more basic arousal process in which the awake patient is able to respond to any stimulus in the environment. The alert but inattentive patient will be attracted to any novel sound, movement, or event occurring in the vicinity; the attentive patient is able to screen out irrelevant stimuli. Attention presupposes alertness, but alertness does not necessarily imply attentiveness.

Vigilance (concentration) is a term that refers to the ability to sustain attention over an extended period of time. This capacity to concentrate is very important for performing intellectual endeavors and may be impaired in both organic and emotional disorders. The concept of inattention (distractibility) is applied to two distinct clinical situations. The first refers to the patient who is clinically inattentive or is unable to sustain sufficient attention to succeed in the simple tests of attention discussed below. The second type of inattention is a specific inattention to stimuli on the side of the body opposite to a unilateral brain lesion. This inattention can be so extreme that the patient becomes unaware of people approaching on the inattentive side (neglect).

# EVALUATION

## Observation

Alertness has been previously evaluated during the portion of the mental status examination that concerned levels of consciousness (see Chapter 3). Considerable information regarding the patient's general attentiveness may be obtained by merely observing the patient's behavior and noting any evidence of distractibility or difficulty in attending to the examiner.

## History

A patient who is having difficulty concentrating on work or other routine tasks is usually able to tell the examiner about the problem. A simple inquiry as to the patient's ability to concentrate or to sustain attention may provide revealing data.

## Digit Repetition

The patient's basic level of attention can be readily assessed by utilizing the digit repetition test. Adequate performance on this task ensures that the patient is able to attend to a verbal stimulus and to sustain attention for the period of time required to repeat the digits. In patients with a significant language disorder (aphasia), this task and the "A" test for vigilance cannot be validly used to assess attention.

*Directions.* Tell the patient, "I am going to say some simple numbers. Listen carefully, and when I am finished, say the numbers after me." Present the digits in a normal tone of voice at a rate of one digit per second. Take care not to group digits either in pairs (e.g., 2 – 6, 5 – 9) or in sequences that could serve as an aid to repetition (e.g., in telephone number form, 376 – 8439). Numbers should be presented randomly without natural sequences (e.g., not 2 – 4 – 6 – 8). Begin with a two-number sequence, and continue until the patient fails.

*Test Items*

| | |
|---|---|
| 3 – 7 | 9 – 2 |
| 7 – 4 – 9 | 1 – 7 – 4 |
| 8 – 5 – 2 – 7 | 5 – 2 – 9 – 7 |
| 2 – 9 – 6 – 8 – 3 | 6 – 3 – 8 – 5 – 1 |
| 5 – 7 – 2 – 9 – 4 – 6 | 2 – 9 – 4 – 7 – 3 – 8 |
| 8 – 1 – 5 – 9 – 3 – 6 – 2 | 4 – 1 – 9 – 2 – 7 – 5 – 1 |
| 3 – 9 – 8 – 2 – 5 – 1 – 4 – 7 | 8 – 5 – 3 – 9 – 1 – 6 – 2 – 7 |
| 7 – 2 – 8 – 5 – 4 – 6 – 7 – 3 – 9 | 2 – 1 – 9 – 7 – 3 – 5 – 8 – 4 – 6 |

*Scoring.* The patient of average intelligence can repeat five to seven digits without difficulty. Repetition of less than five digits by a non-retarded patient without obvious aphasia indicates defective attention.

## Vigilance

A simple test of vigilance that can be readily administered at the bedside is the random letter test. This test consists of a series of random letters among which a target letter appears with greater than random frequency. The patient is required to indicate whenever the target letter is spoken by the examiner.

*Directions.* Tell the patient, "I am going to read you a long series of letters. Whenever you hear the letter A, indicate by tapping the desk." Read the following letter list in a normal tone at a rate of one letter per second.

*Test Items*

L T P E A O A I C T D A L A A

A N I A B F S A M R Z E O A D

P A K L A U C J T O E A B A A

Z Y F M U S A H E V A A R A T

*Scoring.* There are currently only preliminary standardized norms for this test. The average person should complete the task without error ($\bar{x} = 0.2$); a sample of randomly selected brain-damaged patients made an average of 10 errors.[10] Examples of common organic errors are (1) failure to indicate when the target letter has been presented (omission error), (2) indication made when a nontarget letter has been presented (commission error), and (3) failure to stop tapping with the presentation of subsequent nontarget letters (perseveration error).

The serial sevens subtraction test (e.g., counting backward from 100 by sevens: 100 – 93 – 86 . . .) has been traditionally included in mental status examinations. Studies of performance by normal people suggest that errors may reflect premorbid intellectual capability, education, calculating ability, or socioeconomic status, rather than indicating a pathologic process.[11]

## Inattention

Unilateral inattention (suppression or extinction) should be tested during the routine sensory examination by utilizing double (bilateral) simultaneous stimulation.

*Directions.* Double simultaneous stimulation is tested in all major sensory modalities. In tactile testing, corresponding points on both sides of the body are touched simultaneously with equal intensity. Visual testing is done by having the patient face the examiner and fix his or her gaze at a point on the examiner's face. The examiner then moves his or her fingers in both right and left peripheral fields. Auditory testing is carried out by having the examiner stand behind the patient and provide a stimulus of equal intensity to each ear.

Before undertaking bilateral simultaneous stimulation, the examiner must ensure that sensation for each modality is intact bilaterally. If one side is inferior on unilateral testing, defects found during simultaneous testing would not necessarily reflect inattention.

Extinction is present when the patient suppresses the stimuli from one side of the body. Extinction may occur in all modalities (polymodal neglect) or may be restricted to a single modality. When extinction is elicited, the degree of inattention can be assessed by increasing the magnitude of the stimulus on the inattentive side.

When the double simultaneous stimulation includes one proximal and one distal stimulus, the distal stimulus tends to be extinguished.[1] This is particularly true when the proximal stimulus is the face and the distal one is the hand. Normal adults who are under 65 years of age often extinguish the hand stimulus on the first trial, but they will usually begin to identify both stimuli after several trials. Patients with organic brain syndromes rarely recognize the hand stimulus even after as many as 10 trials. This test (face-hand test)[2] is a very useful simple test for organic disease. Some normal elderly individuals will also extinguish the hand stimulus; therefore, the test must be interpreted with caution in patients over 65.

## ANATOMY AND CLINICAL IMPLICATIONS

The basic anatomic structures that are responsible for maintaining an alert state are the brain stem reticular activating system and the diffuse thalamic projection system (the diencephalic extension of the reticular formation).[7]

The mechanism by which this ascending activation is focused and extraneous stimuli are screened out is less certain. Cortical and limbic stimulation can definitely influence the ascending system, so it is probable that attention results from a balance between ascending (reticulocortical) activation and cortical (corticoreticular) modulation.[7] The importance of cortical influence in focusing attention is demonstrated in the experience of every student. Concentration while studying frequently requires conscious voluntary effort; this effort is cortical in origin (probably widespread). The limbic system is also an integral part of the attention process; limbic input adds emotional importance to the object of attention. The child who is watching a cartoon and the adult who is watching an X-rated movie are stimulated to attention by the pleasure and excitement that are being generated by the spectacle. The student who is studying for a test is aided in the need to concentrate by a fear of failure or a drive to succeed. These limbic influences are important and may be the critical factor that facilitates the screening out of extraneous stimuli. The principal stimulus is of greater emotional value than the incidental events in the environment and therefore attracts greater attention.

Since attention represents a complex interaction of limbic, neocortical, and ascending activating functions, there are many areas of the brain in which damage can disrupt the ability to attend. Damage to the ascending activating system itself usually causes alterations in the level of consciousness. In such patients, alterations in attention are directly related to the more basic deficit in alertness. Inattention caused by lesions in the midbrain activating system is probably clinically rare, although a rather profound unilateral inattention has been experimentally produced in monkeys with lesions in the midbrain.[12] Inattention has also been observed clinically in patients with lesions of the thalamus,[13] the posterior internal capsule,[4] and other subcortical structures.[8]

Some of the patients who survived the encephalitis epidemic of 1918 to 1921, which was associated with von Economo's influenza, were left with lesions in the reticular substance of the pons and medulla. These patients developed a behavior pattern characterized by hyperactivity and distractibility that was called "organic driveness."[6] This state is clinically similar to that seen in some hyperactive children.

Probably the most common cause of decreased attention and vigilance in a hospital population is diffuse brain dysfunction. This dysfunction is usually caused by metabolic disturbance, drug intoxication, postsurgical states, or systemic infection. In these confusional states, all cells in the central nervous system are affected. Another common cause of inattention is extensive bilateral cortical damage of any etiology (e.g., atrophy, multiple infarcts, encephalitis, or head trauma). Patients with advanced cortical disease are inattentive and extremely distractible. Any new stimulus in the vicinity will quickly draw their attention; they become "stimulus bound" and are unable to screen out irrelevant stimuli. The cortical role in focusing and maintaining attention is best illustrated in such patients.

Patients with bilateral lesions of the frontal lobes or the limbic system (e.g., Korsakoff's syndrome) have a type of inattention that is characterized by indifference and perseveration. Clinically, they are apathetic toward their surroundings. Test items, per se, have no particular interest to them. Such patients usually perform well on the digit repetition task, but they will not accurately complete the random letter test. These patients will often omit an A at the end of a long sequence (e.g., U C J T O E A) because their attention has wandered. Patients with a frontal lobe lesion also have great difficulty shifting from one pattern of response to another; this deficit results in perseveration. This perseveration is commonly seen both behaviorally and on the random letter test. The series E V A A R A T may be failed in the following way (italic letters indicate the patient's taps) E V *A A R A T*.

Right-hemisphere lesions have a stronger effect upon attention than do left-sided lesions. Denial, unilateral neglect, and extinction on double simultaneous stimulation are more frequent and prominent with right-hemisphere lesions.[5,9] The reason for this peculiar quality of the right hemisphere is not known. It is possible that reticulocortical or corticoreticular fibers are more dense in the right hemisphere, although there is no currently available pathologic evidence that this is true. For a thorough discussion of the theories of the inattention syndrome, see Weinstein and Friedland.[14]

Contralateral inattention to double simultaneous stimulation is seen with parietal lesions of either hemisphere. The damage to parietal tissue apparently reduces reticulocortical interaction on the damaged side, thus allowing the intact hemisphere an advantage in the stimulus rivalry.[3]

There are many functional mood alterations that can affect attention. Anxiety causes distractibility and difficulty concentrating; depression produces disinterest and reduced arousal. All such mood changes will hinder performance on attention tasks and will generally decrease attention.

## SUMMARY

Attention is an interplay among brain stem, limbic activity, and cortical activity that allows the patient to focus on a specific task to the exclusion of irrelevant stimuli. Both functional and organic illness can disrupt attention and cause a failure of vigilance. Assessment of attention must be done early in the mental status examination because the testing of many subsequent functions relies on its integrity.

# REFERENCES

1. Gritchley, M.: The Parietal Lobes. Edward Arnold & Co, London, 1953.
2. Bender, M. B.: Perceptual interactions. In Williams, D. (ed.): Modern Trends in Neurology, Vol. 5. Appleton-Century-Crofts, New York, 1970, pp. 1–28.
3. Denny-Brown, D., Meyers, J., and Hornstein, S.: The significance of perceptual rivalry resulting from parietal lesions. Brain 75:433, 1952.
4. Ferro, J. and Kertesz, A.: Posterior internal capsule infarction associated with neglect. Arch Neurol 41:422, 1984.
5. Gainotti, G.: Emotional behavior and hemispheric side of lesion. Cortex 8:41, 1972.
6. Kahn, E. and Cohen, L.: Organic driveness: A brainstem syndrome and an experience. N Engl J Med 210:748, 1934.
7. Magoun, H.: The Waking Brain. Charles C Thomas, Springfield, Ill., 1963.
8. Mesulum, M. M.: A cortical network for directed attention and unilateral neglect. Ann Neurol 10:309, 1981.
9. Oxbury, J., Campbell, D., and Oxbury, S.: Unilateral spatial neglect and impairment of spatial analysis and perception. Brain 97:551, 1974.
10. Simpson, N. and Black, F. W.: Comparative clinical utility of the Wechsler Memory Scale and the Strub-Black Mental Status Examination with neurologically impaired patients. Paper presented at the 30th Annual Convention of the Southeastern Psychological Association, New Orleans, March 1984.
11. Smith, A.: The serial sevens subtraction test. Arch Neurol 17:18, 1976.
12. Watson, R. T., et al: Neglect after mesenaphalic reticular formation lesions. Neurology 24:294, 1974.
13. Watson, R. T., Valenstein, E., and Heilman, K. M.: Thalamic neglect. Arch Neurol 38:501, 1981.
14. Weinstein, E. A. and Friedland, R. P. (eds.): Hemi-Inattention and Hemispheric Specialization. Advances in Neurology, Vol. 18. Raven Press, New York, 1977.

# CHAPTER 5

# Language

Language is the basic tool of human communication and is crucial in assessing most cognitive abilities. Therefore, its integrity must be established early in the course of mental status testing. If deficits are found in the language system, the subsequent evaluation of cognitive factors such as verbal memory, proverb interpretation, and oral calculations becomes difficult, if not impossible.

Language disturbances are commonly seen in patients with focal or diffuse brain disease; in fact, demonstration of a specific language disturbance is pathognomonic of brain damage. Language disturbances have been well studied, and a number of distinct clinical neuroanatomic syndromes have been described. These are of importance to the clinician because of the relationship of specific language syndromes with neuroanatomic lesions. The ability to communicate using language is critical to the patient, and any disruption of this ability will result in a significant handicap in day-to-day living.

The examiner must develop a systematic approach to language evaluation and must become acquainted with the various classic language syndromes. Cerebral vascular accidents (strokes), brain tumors, trauma, and other lesions cause a variety of language disturbances. These disturbances are not always easily characterized by a cursory examination. A familiarity with testing and the patterns of language disruption will make the aphasias, alexias, and agraphias more understandable.

## TERMINOLOGY

*Dysarthria* refers to a specific disorder of articulation in which basic language (grammar, comprehension, and word choice) is intact. Patients with pure dysarthria produce distorted speech sounds that cannot be accurately transcribed by a listener. The speech can be unintelligible and may not resemble English speech sounds.

*Dysprosody* is an interruption of speech melody. Speech inflection and rhythm are disturbed. The resulting speech production can be monotonal, halting, and can at times mimic a foreign accent.

Buccofacial or oral *apraxia* is the inability to perform skilled movements of the face and speech apparatus in the presence of normal comprehension, muscle strength, and coordination. When asked to show how they would blow out a match, apraxic patients may have difficulty approximating a pucker, may inhale instead of exhale vigorously without puckering their lips, or may merely say the word "blow." Any of these errors would be classified as apraxic. At times, this oral apraxia is evident as the patient attempts to produce speech sounds; this is referred to as verbal apraxia.

*Aphasia* is a true language disturbance in which the patient produces errors of grammar and word choice or has a defect in comprehension. The basic aphasic defect is in higher integrative language processing, although articulation and praxic errors may be present. Aphasia usually refers to a loss of language after brain damage, but the term developmental aphasia is used when a child has a specific delay in language acquisition disproportionate to general cognitive development.

*Alexia* is the term used to describe a loss of reading ability in a previously literate person. Alexia does not refer only to a total loss of reading ability, but to any level of disturbance in reading. Alexia is not synonymous with dyslexia. Dyslexia refers to a specific developmental learning disorder of children who have normal intelligence, yet experience unusual difficulty in learning to read.

*Agraphia* is an acquired disturbance in writing. It refers specifically to errors of language and not to problems with the actual formation of letters or poor handwriting.

## EVALUATION

The evaluation of the language system should be performed in an orderly fashion. Specific attention must be paid to spontaneous speech, comprehension, repetition, and naming. Reading and writing should be assessed after verbal language has been evaluated. A short period of systematic testing can usually identify and roughly characterize an aphasic deficit. The aphasic patient is always agraphic and is frequently alexic; accordingly, in these cases, the testing of reading and writing may be abbreviated. In the nonaphasic patient, reading and writing should be fully evaluated because alexia and/or agraphia may be seen in isolation. Language testing can be very comprehensive; for further information, the interested examiner is referred to the test batteries listed in Appendix 1.

## Handedness

Handedness and cerebral dominance for language are closely allied; therefore, the patient's handedness should be determined prior to language testing. First, ask the patient whether he or she is right- or left-handed. Many natural left-handers have been taught to write with the right hand. Accordingly, observation of the hand used for writing may not be an accurate reflection of natural handedness. Next, ask the patient which hand he or she uses to hold a knife, throw a ball, stir coffee, and flip a coin. Also, ask the patient if he or she has any tendency to use the opposite hand for any skilled movement. In addition, a family history of left-handedness or ambidexterity is important, since cerebral dominance for language is significantly influenced by heredity. There is a spectrum of handedness that ranges from strong right-handedness to left-handedness. Unilateral handedness tends to be much stronger in right-handed individuals than in left. Patients with a strong family history of left-handedness tend to be ambidextrous.[20] A statement of the patient's handedness as well as the family history should be recorded.

## Spontaneous Speech

The first step in language testing is to listen carefully to the patient's spontaneous speech. If the patient offers none, certain open-ended questions should be asked in order to elicit speech production. Listening to the patient's spontaneous speech for even a brief period of time may provide invaluable information that cannot be obtained during more formal aspects of the language examination. It is wise to ask relatively uncomplicated questions, such as "Tell me why you are in the hospital" or "Tell me a bit about your work." This type of general conversational question affords the patient a familiar topic and usually elicits his or her best efforts. In contrast, questions that require a mere "yes" or "no" answer will not provide sufficient speech output for evaluation. Pictures may be used to stimulate speech; however, they can restrict language output because of the limitations of the specific stimulus.

Several observations must be made while listening to the patient's spontaneous speech. First, is speech output present? Second, is the speech dysarthric or dysprosodic? Third, is there evidence of specific aphasic errors? The most obviously abnormal output is the total lack of any speech. These patients may make some vocalizations but no meaningful linguistic utterances. This reduced output may be due to a severe dysarthria, apraxia (buccofacial), or a true aphasia. Next in severity is a specific aphasic disorder that is characterized by stereotyped output in which the patient repeats the same utterance in response to each question. The utterance is usually a nonsense word like "bica, bica" or "a dis, a dis, a dis." Patients with very restricted output can, however, often surprise the naive examiner by producing well-articulated curse words or short phrases under emotional stress.

Aphasic language production is characterized by errors of grammatical structure, difficulty in word finding, and the presence of word substitutions (paraphasias). One common type of aphasic speech pattern has been classified as nonfluent.[3,15] Nonfluent output is sparse, effortful, contains primarily nouns (substantive words), is agrammatic, and contains frequent word-finding pauses. For instance, the nonfluent patient describing winter weather might say, "ah, ah, chold ... snow ... frezing ... ah, ah ... cold." At the other end of the spectrum of fluency is a group of aphasic patients who produce an easily flowing speech that is remarkably empty of content and contains many abnormal words (paraphasias). Paraphasias are words that are either substitutions for the correct word (e.g., "I drove home in my pen") or contain substituted syllables (e.g., "I drove home in my lar"). The complete word substitution ("pen" for "car") is a verbal or semantic paraphasia. The syllable substitution ("lar" for "car") is a phonemic or literal paraphasia. A third variety of paraphasia is the neologistic (new word) paraphasia, which is a completely non-English word substitution (e.g., "I drove home in my strub"). Fluent aphasic speech is an easily recognizable speech pattern. The output is fluent and is characterized by normal or excessive rate of word production, often with a distinct press of speech (rapid pressure to speak). Content words (nouns and verbs) are lacking; and in contradistinction to nonfluent output, small grammatical words such as articles, conjunctions, and interjections prevail. The nouns and verbs are often paraphasic. Because of the difficulty in producing nouns, word-finding pauses may interrupt the easy flow of speech. A fluent aphasic who was describing a picture of a man after a shipwreck said the following: "It is a ... I can see it ... it is near a cold and he has a ... actually what has happened is part of a ... the rest of it there is a man right here and he is cold being out there." Occasionally, the language of the aphasic contains so many paraphasic errors that the discourse is virtually unintelligible and impossible to follow. The term jargon aphasia is used for this heavily paraphasic but fluent speech.

The expressive language of many aphasics cannot be strictly classified according to fluency but, rather, is a mixture. The primary goal for the student who is evaluating a brain-damaged patient is to recognize that the language production is aphasic. With experience, the examiner will be able to accurately recognize aphasic language and to classify the patient's language output. The classification of language output often gives important information as to the locus of the brain lesion. Patients with nonfluent aphasia are likely to have an anterior left-hemisphere lesion; whereas patients with fluent aphasia usually have posterior lesions.[3] The classification of an aphasia does not rest upon the output characteristics alone; a full language evaluation is always indicated.

## Verbal Fluency

Verbal fluency refers to the ability to produce spontaneous speech fluently without undue word-finding pauses or failures in word searching. Normal speech requires verbal fluency in the production of responses and the formulation of spontaneous conversational speech. This ability is often impaired after brain injury, especially with anterior left-hemisphere lesions. Aphasic patients will almost invariably demonstrate impaired fluency on formal testing. Additionally, individuals with relatively normal expressive speech and no other signs of word-finding difficulty may show subtle deficits on fluency tests. Thus, verbal fluency can be considered a high level of word-finding efficiency which may detect mild language problems due to left-hemisphere lesions or early dementias that do not produce frank aphasia.

Verbal fluency is typically evaluated by tabulating the number of words the patient produces within a restricted category (e.g., "animals" or words beginning with the "letter A") and time limit. Two easily administered techniques are the "Animal Naming Test"[19] and the "FAS" (controlled oral word association) test.[7]

*Directions:* For animal naming, instruct the patient to recall and name as many animals as possible. Any animal from the zoo, the farm, the jungle, the water, or the house is acceptable. Time the patient's performance for 90 seconds, encouraging him or her to continue whenever necessary. The score is the number of correctly produced animal names during the patient's best 60 seconds. Record the correct responses as well as any paraphasic productions.

The normal individual should produce from 18 to 22 animal names during a 60-second period, with the expected variation being ±5–7.[19,33] Scores below 13 in otherwise normal patients should raise the question of impaired naming; scores below 10 are highly indicative of a word-finding problem.

The FAS test consists of three separate timed word-naming trials, using the letters F, A, and S, respectively. The patient is instructed to name as many words as possible that begin with the stipulated letter during a 60-second trial. Record the patient's responses, including paraphasic and repeated words, that were produced in the three 60-second trials. Normal people name from 36 to 60 words, with performance depending on both age and educational level.[7] An inability to name 12 or more words per letter is indicative of reduced verbal fluency. Performance on this test should be cautiously interpreted in patients with less than 10 years of formal education.

## Comprehension

Assessment of the comprehension of spoken language is the next step in the language evaluation. Comprehension must be tested in a structured fashion without reliance upon the patient's ability to answer verbally. The most common error is to ask the patient to answer general or open-ended questions. Such questions require the patient to construct complex verbal answers that test the integrity of the entire language system and not verbal comprehension in isolation. Comprehension testing should require the minimum verbal response necessary for the patient to demonstrate that he or she has understood the examiner. For example, asking the patient to answer the question "What was the weather like in January?" does not assess language comprehension in isolation; whereas questions such as "Is it snowing out today?" do.

We use two methods of testing comprehension: pointing commands and questions that can be answered with a yes or no response. Pointing to single objects in the room, body parts, or articles collected from the examiner's pockets (e.g., coins, comb, pencil, key, and so forth) is an excellent way to quantify single-word comprehension. This task may be increased in complexity by requiring that the patient point to an increasing number of objects in sequence. Increase the number of objects until the patient consistently fails. The patient of average intelligence without aphasia should succeed in pointing to four objects or more. The aphasic patient with comprehension difficulty may be able to accurately point to one or two items; therefore, it is important to continue testing until a point of consistent failure is reached. This test provides an evaluation of single-word comprehension, auditory retention, and sequence memory. For clarity, the level of performance should be accurately described on the test form.

Next, a series of simple and complex questions that require only "yes" or "no" answers should be asked. For example: "Is this a hotel?" "Is it raining today?" "Do you eat breakfast before dinner?" Material may be as simple or complex as necessary. Before testing, be sure that the patient can reliably indicate "yes" and "no." Many patients will confuse these two items and be unable to accurately speak or nod appropriately.

Also, it is important to ask at least six questions, since correct responses can occur by chance alone 50 percent of the time with yes/no questions. Correct answers should alternate from yes to no randomly because brain-damaged patients tend to perseverate. It is not uncommon for a patient to answer "yes" to 10 consecutive questions without knowing the correct answer to any of the questions.

Many clinicians test comprehension by asking patients to carry out motor commands such as "Show me how to light a cigarette" or "Stick out your tongue." If the patient correctly carries ou t such commands, he or she has certainly understood them; however, n any aphasic patients have significant apraxia and fail to follow the cummand because of a high-level motor problem and not because of poor verbal comprehension. For this reason, verbal commands must be used with caution.

## Repetition

Repetition of spoken language is linguistically and, to some extent, anatomically a distinct function. Therefore, it is clinically relevant to test it specifically. There are certain types of aphasia in which repetition may be either spared or involved exclusively. Repetition is a complex process that can be affected by impaired auditory processing, disturbed speech production, or disconnection between the receptive and expressive language functions.

Testing should be done with material of ascending difficulty. Start with single monosyllabic words and proceed to complex sentences. The following list of items provides a range of difficulty. The patient should be asked to repeat the word or sentence after the examiner.

1. Ball
2. Help
3. Airplane
4. Hospital
5. Mississippi River
6. The little boy went home.
7. We all went over there together.
8. The old car wouldn't start on Tuesday morning.
9. The fat short boy dropped the china vase.
10. Each fight readied the boxer for the championship bout.

The examiner must listen for paraphasias, grammatical errors, omissions, and additions. Normal people and nonaphasic brain-damaged patients can accurately repeat sentences of 19 syllables.[30] Performance is related to intelligence and educational level; however, errorless performance is expected on these items.

## Naming and Word Finding

The ability to name objects is one of the earliest acquired and most basic language functions. It is also almost invariably disturbed in all types of aphasias.[19] Word-finding difficulty is closely related to impaired naming ability (anomia) and refers to a reduced availability of the nouns and verbs used in spontaneous speech. Specific word-finding problems can be detected by listening to the aphasic patient's spontaneous speech. Asking the patient to describe a picture that contains objects and actions will dramatize the word-finding defect. Anomia is best assessed by confrontation naming. In this task, the examiner points to a variety of objects and asks the patient to name them. The examiner should select from 10 to 20 items. Several categories of objects should be used (colors, body parts, room objects, articles of clothing, and parts of objects). Various categories are chosen because some aphasic patients have a curious inability to name objects in a specific category, while maintaining adequate ability to name objects in other categories. Since the disruption of naming has varying degrees of severity, it is important to use uncommon (low frequency of usage) items as well as common (high frequency of usage) items. For example, "nose," "arm," and "floor" are common, high-frequency, words; whereas "watch crystal," "shin," and "coat lapel" are uncommon, low-frequency, words. Many aphasic patients will be able to quickly and accurately name common objects, only to show great hesitancy, paraphasia, and circumlocution with uncommon objects. Some patients obviously recognize the object and are able to demonstrate and describe its use, but cannot name it. For example, a patient shown a door key responded with "oh, you know ... the thing used to get in the ... you turn it to get in."

The 20 items in Table 5-1, listed in ascending order of difficulty, are suggested for evaluating naming ability. The examiner should note that the labels for parts of objects are less frequently used in expressive speech; accordingly, most aphasic patients will have relatively more difficulty with this category. With experience, the examiner may develop a personal repertoire of items tailored to his or her own office and patient population.

## Reading

Reading ability is one of the few aspects of mental status testing that is directly related to educational experience. It is important, therefore, to determine the patient's educational background before testing reading. Demonstrating an alexia (reading deficit) in a patient only to dis-

TABLE 5-1. Objects for Confrontation Naming in Ascending Order of Difficulty by Category

| Colors | Body Parts |
| --- | --- |
| Red | Eye |
| Blue | Leg |
| Yellow | Teeth |
| Pink | Thumb |
| Purple | Knuckles |

| Clothing and Room Objects | Parts of Objects |
| --- | --- |
| Door | Watch stem (winder) |
| Watch | Coat lapel |
| Shoe | Watch crystal (lens) |
| Shirt | Sole of shoe |
| Ceiling | Buckle of belt |

cover that he or she has had but 3 years of formal education is merely documenting the patient's illiteracy.

Both reading comprehension and reading aloud should be tested. Both are usually defective in the same patient, but either can be disturbed in isolation. If the patient is not aphasic, screen for alexia by having the patient read a paragraph from a newspaper or magazine. Testing reading in the aphasic patient should begin with short single words, then phrases, sentences, and finally paragraphs. First, have the patient read the item aloud, and then have him or her indicate comprehension by pointing to the object or saying or nodding "yes" or "no." For example, if the patient read the sentence "The boy and girl walked in the snow," the examiner could ask, "Did the boy go alone?" or "Was it raining when the boy and girl went for a walk?"

The examiner should note any syllable or word substitutions (paralexic errors), omitted words, and defects in comprehension. Occasionally, patients have visual field defects or problems in ocular motility. In such cases, the examiner must assist the patient in staying on the written line and ensure that the patient completes one line before starting another. By careful observation and examination, the examiner can readily separate the true alexias from problems with the mechanics of reading.

## Writing

Writing must be tested in the same careful way as was reading. If the patient shows evidence of aphasia, he or she will undoubtedly have an agraphia. First, have the patient write letters and numbers to dictation. Next, ask the patient to write the names of common objects or body parts. Third, if the patient can successfully write single words, ask him or her to write a short sentence describing the weather, his or her job, or a picture from a magazine. Asking the patient to write his or her name is not always useful, since name writing may be preserved even in the presence of gross agraphia. In the literate nonaphasic patient, the examination can begin with this sentence-writing task. Writing to dictation is a somewhat different task that can also be tested if time allows. The aphasic patient who is unable to write spontaneously may show residual writing ability when asked to write to dictation.

Agraphia is diagnosed when basic language errors, gross spelling errors, or paragraphias (word or syllable substitutions) are present.

Writing can often show a misalignment, in which the written line slants upward. This misalignment is an error in the mechanics of writing, but is not an agraphia, per se.

## Spelling

Spelling is a complex, little studied higher-language function that is strongly associated with educational experience. For practical purposes, spelling can be evaluated by asking the patient to spell dictated words aloud and then to write them. Gross errors in spelling can be detected in bedside testing; if it is important to establish an actual level of competence, standardized achievement tests can be used (see Appendix 1).

# CLINICAL IMPLICATIONS

## Cerebral Dominance

Approximately 90 percent of the population is considered definitely right-handed. Of this 90 percent, more than 99 percent are strongly left-hemisphere dominant for language.[5] Because of this strong language dominance in right-handed individuals, left-hemisphere lesions will frequently cause aphasia; whereas right-hemisphere lesions rarely result in such deficits (i.e., a crossed aphasia).[34] Left-handed individuals have a far different pattern of cerebral dominance for language. Eighty percent have some degree of language representation in both hemispheres.[17] In individuals with a strong family history of left-handedness (sinistrality), this mixed dominance tends to be more prominent. Strongly left-handed individuals with no history of familial sinistrality tend to have the strongest left-hemisphere dominance for language of all left-handed individuals. Accordingly, damage to either hemisphere in a left-handed patient will result in aphasia in 80 percent of all cases. The aphasia will be less severe than that resulting from a similar lesion in the left hemisphere in a right-handed patient. Knowing the patient's dominance for language is important for localizing lesions and for deciding the risk to language of neurosurgical procedures. In cases in which documentation of hemispheric dominance for language is critical (e.g., left-handed patient with a right middle cerebral artery aneurysm), an intracarotid Amytal injection at the time of angiography can often establish dominance.[32]

## Aphasia Syndromes

The impairment of language secondary to brain damage is not a unitary process; all components of language can show variable disruption. The extensive study of right-handed aphasic patients has resulted in a generally accepted schema of cortical localization of language. Since there are overlapping features among aphasic patients who demonstrate a picture of mixed aphasia, some aphasiologists do not feel that this traditional neurologic classification is suitable for neurolinguistic research.[9] However, this classification system follows the classic anatomic pattern, is easy for the student to understand, and is useful for the clinician for localizing lesions.

The posterior language area (area 1, Fig. 5-1) is the cortical area primarily concerned with the comprehension of spoken language. This area has classically been referred to as Wernicke's area, although the exact boundaries of the region have not been agreed upon.[6] The anterior language area (area 2, Fig. 5-1) subsumes the functions of language production. Brodmann's area 44 within the anterior language area is the classic Broca's area. Traditionally, patients with damage in the posterior speech area are called receptive aphasics because of their primary difficulty in understanding spoken language. Patients with lesions in the anterior area are called expressive aphasics because of their difficulty in producing language. The problem in using the term "expressive aphasia" is that all aphasics have some type of abnormal language expression; thus, the inexperienced examiner tends to classify all aphasias as "expressive aphasia." For this reason, we prefer to use the classification system described below rather than the expressive-receptive dichotomy. The clinical features of a patient's aphasia change dramatically over time. The acute destructive lesion causes maximal language disruption and is often associated with considerable disorientation and confusion. In the first few weeks, recovery is rapid and the aphasic picture constantly changes. After 3 weeks, the aphasic pattern is more stable and may be fully assessed. The final prognosis of language recovery, however, cannot be given at that time because the recovery process can continue for months or even years.

FIGURE 5-1. Anterior and posterior language areas.

## Global Aphasia

Global aphasia is the most common and severe form of aphasia. It is characterized by spontaneous speech that is either absent or reduced to a few stereotyped words or sounds (e.g., "ba, ba, ba" or "dis, a dis, a dis"). Comprehension is absent or reduced to only recognition of the patient's name or a few selected words. Performance on repetition is at the same level as spontaneous speech. Reading and writing are likewise severely impaired. Global aphasia is caused by a large lesion that damages most or all of the combined language areas 1 and 2. The most common lesion is an occlusion of the internal carotid artery or the middle cerebral artery at its origin. Unfortunately, the prognosis is poor for language recovery in these patients. Global aphasia is almost always associated with hemiplegia. Because of these combined deficits, such patients have a severe chronic disability.

## Broca's Aphasia

This classic syndrome has as its hallmark nonfluent, dysarthric, effortful speech. The patient utters mostly nouns and verbs (high-content words), with a paucity of grammatical fillers. The characteristic speech has been called agrammatic or telegraphic. For example, one Broca's aphasic patient described a picture of a boy on a stool stealing cookies while his mother is washing dishes and letting the sink run over[19] in the following manner: "Boy . . . ah girl steal cookie. . . . Stool falling water spilling. . . . Dishes." Repetition and reading aloud are as severely impaired in these patients as is their spontaneous speech. Auditory and reading comprehension are surprisingly intact, although the comprehension of complex grammatical phrases (e.g., "Do you eat lunch before breakfast?") is often impaired. Naming may show occasional paraphasias.

This characteristic nonfluent aphasic syndrome results from a lesion in the anterior speech area (area 2, Fig. 5-1). The lesion causing Broca's aphasia includes more than area 44 alone. Lesions restricted exclusively to area 44 result in only transient dysarthria or dysprosody.[23] Auditory and visual (reading) comprehension are intact because parietal and temporal lobes are not damaged. The Broca's aphasic patient usually has a right hemiplegia.

These patients often have an interesting and significant emotional change, characterized by frustration, agitation, and depression.[4] Whether this emotional change is a functional reaction to the loss of speech or a specific organic change associated with left frontal lobe damage is not yet known.[29]

The prognosis for language recovery in Broca's aphasia is generally more favorable than in global aphasia. Because of intact comprehension, these patients adjust better to life situations.

Wernicke's Aphasia

Wernicke's aphasia can be considered the linguistic opposite of Broca's aphasia. The patient with Wernicke's aphasia has fluent, effortless, well-articulated speech. The output, however, contains many paraphasias and is often devoid of substantive words. There is often a great press to speak. The following is an example of speech in Wernicke's aphasia. The patient was a ferry boat captain with a left temporal lobe brain tumor. In describing his previous work, the patient said, "Yea, I walked on the . . . always over . . . then pull it in . . . tie the . . . ah, ah over and back over wellendy catch it. . . . " The spontaneous speech can range from comprehensive sentences with occasional paraphasic errors to totally incomprehensible jargon in which most words are paraphasias and the output is empty and devoid of content.

The essential feature of Wernicke's aphasia is a severe disturbance of auditory comprehension. Because the comprehension defect is so marked, the patients answer questions inappropriately and are completely unaware that their answers are often total nonsense. Repetition is severely impaired because of a severe auditory processing defect. Naming is grossly paraphasic. Reading and writing are also markedly impaired.

The lesion that causes Wernicke's aphasia is in the posterior language area (area 1, Fig. 5-1). The more severe the defect in auditory comprehension, the more likely it is that the lesion involves the posterior portion of the superior temporal gyrus. If single-word comprehension is good, yet comprehension of complex material is impaired, the lesion is more likely to involve the parietal lobe rather than the superior temporal lobe.[19] Since the damage is restricted to parietal and temporal lobes, the classic Wernicke's aphasic patient does not have a hemiplegia.

The Wernicke's aphasic patient is often initially considered to be psychotic rather than aphasic by family and medical personnel alike. This confusion arises because the patient usually does not have a hemiplegia and produces inappropriate, but often reasonably well formed, sentences. The gross comprehension deficit is not appreciated, and the inappropriate answers to the examiner's questions are judged to be due to a basic thought disorder rather than a language disorder. The patient's brain damage is overlooked because of the absence of neurologic findings such as hemiparesis, sensory loss, or altered level of consciousness. These patients can often develop unusual behavior patterns. They are frequently totally unaware of their problem and talk endlessly without the slightest appreciation of their language deficit. This indifference may approach the point of euphoria. Other patients, however, develop a pronounced paranoid attitude with combative behavior. This behavioral change may become chronic and require major tranquilization and/or confinement to a psychiatric ward.

Patients with severe comprehension deficits do not have a good prognosis for language recovery, even with intensive language therapy. Milder Wernicke's aphasia may evolve into conduction or anomic aphasia, conditions in which auditory comprehension is adequate, but output contains paraphasias and word-finding pauses.

Conduction Aphasia

Conduction aphasia is characterized by fluent, yet halting, speech with word-finding pauses and literal paraphasias. Comprehension is good, naming is mildly disturbed, and repetition is severely defective. This syndrome demonstrates that repetition and propositional speech (everyday language used to describe events or thoughts) are distinct psycholinguistic processes. In conduction aphasia, reading is quite good, but writing shows errors in spelling, word choice, and syntax.

FIGURE 5-2. Representation of arcuate fasciculus and anterior and posterior language areas.

There are two lesions known to cause this type of aphasia. The first is usually reported as involving the supramarginal gyrus and arcuate fasciculus, a long fiber tract (AF on Fig. 5-2) between the anterior and posterior areas. The second is a lesion that damages the insula, contiguous auditory cortex, and underlying white matter. This lesion spares the arcuate fasciculus, which arches higher into the parietal operculum.[12] This entity represents one of the disconnection syndromes,[14] since it literally disconnects the auditory sensory cortex from the motor speech cortex.

## Anomic Aphasia

There are aphasic patients whose only language defects are word-finding difficulty and an inability to name objects on confrontation.

This condition has been labeled anomic, nominal, or amnesic aphasia. Spontaneous speech is usually fluent and grammatically rich but contains many word-finding pauses. The patients produce paraphasias when searching for specific object names. Auditory comprehension is very good, except when the patient is asked to point to a series of specific objects. This comprehension defect is a result of two-way dissociation of naming: the patient cannot name objects and frequently has difficulty recognizing object names when offered in examination. Repetition is good, with the exception of sentences that contain many nouns. Reading and writing may be impaired in specific patients; the degree of alexia and agraphia depends entirely upon the location of the lesion that is responsible for the aphasia.

Lesions in many parts of the dominant hemisphere can cause anomic aphasia; thus, the localizing significance of this type of aphasia is limited. The most severe anomic aphasia, however, is noted in patients with temporal lobe lesions involving the second and third temporal gyri. This area cannot be considered an actual "word dictionary" but includes important pathways from the occipital lobe to the limbic system that are critical for object naming.[14] Lesions in the parietotemporal area also result in rather severe anomia. Patients with these lesions also have substantial alexias with agraphia. Accordingly, the combined syndrome of alexia and agraphia with anomic aphasia will localize a lesion to the left parietotemporal area.

Anomias may be so mild that they are scarcely detectable in normal conversation, while other anomias are sufficiently severe that spontaneous output is nonfluent and empty of meaningful content. The prognosis for language recovery will be dependent upon the severity of the initial defect. Since language output is relatively spared and comprehension is reasonably intact, such patients make better life adjustments than other, more severely affected, aphasic patients.


Transcortical Aphasias

The transcortical aphasias are characterized by intact repetition of spoken language but disruption of other language functions. Some patients will have difficulty producing language, yet have adequate comprehension; others will produce fluent speech, but have poor comprehension.

The patient with transcortical motor aphasia is able to repeat, comprehend, and read well, but has the restricted spontaneous speech of the Broca's aphasic patient. In contrast, the transcortical sensory aphasic patient repeats well but does not comprehend what he or she hears or repeats. Spontaneous speech and naming are fluent but paraphasic, as in Wernicke's aphasia. Occasionally, a patient may have a combination of transcortical motor and sensory aphasias. These patients are able to repeat long sentences, even in a foreign language, with remarkable accuracy. Repetition is very easy to initiate in these patients, even inadvertently, because they have a tendency to be echolalic (to repeat everything said within the range of their hearing).

The lesions that cause transcortical aphasia are extensive, crescent-shaped infarcts within the border zones between major cerebral vessels (e.g., within the frontal lobe between the territories of the anterior and middle cerebral arteries). Transcortical motor aphasia is seen with an anterior border-zone lesion that resembles a reversed C (Fig. 5-3). These lesions spare the superior temporal and inferior frontal cortex (areas 22 and 44 and immediate environs) and the parietal perisylvian cortex. This spared perisylvian cortex is all that is required for complete and accurate language repetition. When this region is the only language area spared by combined border-zone infarcts, the resulting language deficit (echolalia) has been called the isolation of speech syndrome.[16] The most common causes of the transcortical aphasias are as follows: (1) anoxia secondary to decreased cerebral circulation, as seen in cardiac arrest; (2) occlusion or significant stenosis of the carotid artery; (3) anoxia due to carbon monoxide poisoning; and (4) dementia.[28]

FIGURE 5-3. Border-zone infarct that produces transcortical aphasia.

Recovery from transcortical sensory aphasia is relatively good, but little data is available regarding the prognosis in the motor or mixed transcortical aphasias.

### Subcortical Aphasia

Some patients with vascular lesions (either hemorrhage or infarct) of the thalamus, putamen/caudate, or internal capsule will demonstrate aphasic symptoms. They are dysarthric and often run words together. They have mild anomia and comprehension deficits, yet have excellent repetition.[11,24] Anterior lesions tend to produce speech-production problems; posterior lesions result in comprehension difficulty.[25]

The mechanisms by which these subcortical lesions produce aphasia are not clear. In some cases, the disorder seems more a motor-speech problem; in others, a true aphasia or language disturbance is present.[21] Since the cortex is thought to be the repository of language engrams, it is most likely that the subcortical damage alters the input to and the function of the overlying cortex. In a recent study of glucose uptake in subcortical aphasic patients, Metter and associates[22] demonstrated a definite decrease in cortical metabolism in addition to the expected decreased metabolism of the subcortical structures.

### Aphasia in Left-Handed Individuals

Owing to their mixed dominance, the left-handed individual is likely to become aphasic secondary to a lesion in either hemisphere. The resultant aphasia is usually milder and shows greater recovery than does an aphasia due to a similar lesion in a right-handed patient. In 35 to 40 percent of the cases, the aphasia cannot be classified within the traditional scheme. Wernicke's aphasia or the agrammatism of Broca's aphasia are rarely seen. Decreased verbal fluency and dysarthria are common, but comprehension is usually relatively intact. Repetition is relatively spared. Naming and reading are defective when the patient's lesion is in the left hemisphere.[8,18]

## Language in Alzheimer's Disease

A progressive deterioration in language facility is observed in atrophic (cortical) dementia. In the earliest stage, the patient's conversation wanders in a circumlocutory fashion and can be difficult to follow. The content of conversational speech is simplified and reflects the general decrease in intellectual ability. Word-finding pauses are present and verbal fluency is reduced. As the disease progresses, word finding becomes more prominent and paraphasic substitutions are seen. Spontaneous speech lacks relevance and may be tangential. Intrusions of words or phrases from earlier parts of a conversation may appear at inappropriate times. Comprehension is also decreased. Naming is reduced and may be paraphasic. Repetition, however, is preserved quite late in the course of the dementia.

In the late stages of the disease, there is little spontaneous speech or comprehension. Echolalia is often seen. In the final decorticate state, the patients become mute.[1,10]

## Pure Word Deafness

Pure word deafness is a rare syndrome in which patients do not have aphasic speech, agraphia, or alexia, yet have a total lack of comprehension of verbal language. Hearing is intact, and they recognize non-language sounds (auditory gnosis).

The lesion that produces this condition is located in the posterior language area and is usually bilateral. The deep lesion in the temporal lobe disconnects auditory input from the auditory cortex.[2]

## Articulation Disturbances

Pure dysarthrias are caused by lesions in any of the inputs to the muscles of articulation: the cortex, as in Broca's aphasia; the basal ganglia, as in parkinsonism or cerebral palsy; bilateral striatal or pontine lesions, as in pseudobulbar palsy; or the bulbar neurons, as in amyotrophic lateral sclerosis. The patient with pure dysarthria will be able to communicate normally using reading and writing.

Buccofacial apraxia may be caused by various lesions between the supramarginal gyrus and the frontal lobe in the dominant hemisphere. Lesions in these areas appear to interrupt the motor planning necessary for the complex movements of normal speech. Many aphasic patients, particularly those with Broca's or conduction aphasia, have considerable apraxia of facial movement. Some patients with language output resembling Broca's aphasia may, in fact, have pure buccofacial apraxia. The difficulty in separating the aphasic and apraxic components of speech in some patients has resulted in some speech pathologists considering Broca's aphasia as merely a motor-speech disorder and not a true aphasia. Broca's aphasia can be seen, however, in the absence of any buccofacial apraxia. Therefore, careful examination of each patient is important to separate the apraxic and aphasic components.

Dysfluency (stuttering or stammering) is another speech-production problem. This is not an aphasia, an apraxia, or a dysarthria. It is a common speech disorder whose exact etiology is not known. Both organic and functional explanations have been advanced but not proven. Dysfluency may be acquired secondary to a brain lesion, or it may be developmental in nature.

## Alexia

There are several distinct syndromes in which reading ability is impaired by acquired brain lesions. The classic syndrome of pure alexia without agraphia[13,14] is caused by a left posterior cerebral artery occlusion in a right-handed individual. The resulting cerebral infarct damages the posterior portion of the corpus callosum as well as the left occipital lobe. Since the left visual cortex is damaged, all visual information enters only the right hemisphere. The right visual cortex perceives the written material, but is unable to transmit it to the left hemisphere because of the callosal lesion (Fig. 5-4). The inferior parietal lobule in the dominant hemisphere (primarily area 39, the angular gyrus) is the association cortex that combines the visual and auditory information necessary for reading and writing. In alexia without agraphia, the inferior parietal lobule is disconnected from all visual input. Since the lobule and its connections within the language area are intact, the patient is able to write normally. One of the dramatic aspects of this syndrome is the patient's ability to write lengthy, meaningful messages, only to be unable to read his or her own writing. These patients are able to understand words spelled aloud. Interestingly, most patients with this syndrome can name objects and discuss visual events that are occurring in their environment. This type of visual information must cross to the left hemisphere by some pathway other than the damaged posterior corpus callosum.

A second distinct type of alexia results from damage to the inferior parietal lobule itself (angular gyrus and environs). This lesion renders the patient both unable to read and to write. This syndrome is classically called alexia with agraphia. These patients are not appreciably aphasic, but they may have a certain degree of anomia. Recognition of this syndrome is clinically important for localization, as in the right-handed patient, the lesion is invariably in the left inferior parietal area.

The most common acquired alexia is neither of the pure syndromes, but is the alexia that is associated with aphasia.

## Agraphia

Writing is a complex motor task that involves the translation of a language item into written symbols. The linguistic message to be written originates in the posterior language area, is then translated into vi-

FIGURE 5-4. The cross-hatched area represents infarction of the left visual cortex and the posterior portion of the corpus callosum. The visual information from the right visual cortex *(arrow)* is unable to reach the left inferior parietal lobule (39 and 40) because of the callosal lesion.

sual symbols in the inferior parietal area, and is finally sent to the frontal language area for motor processing. Lesions within any of these language areas will cause an agraphia. With the exception of patients with pure word deafness, all aphasic patients show some degree of agraphia. Although the most common agraphia is the form seen with aphasia, there are circumstances in which agraphia may be seen in the absence of aphasia. Two syndromes are seen in patients with damage in the dominant parietal lobe: the first is the agraphia seen with alexia, which was described in the previous section; the second is a syndrome of agraphia in association with other parietal lobe signs (dyscalculia, right-left disorientation, and finger agnosia), called the Gerstmann syndrome. The Gerstmann syndrome is discussed in detail in Chapter 9.

There is a rare pure agraphia that occurs only in the left hand. This syndrome is seen in patients with lesions of the anterior corpus callosum. These patients are agraphic with the left hand only, because the right motor cortex is disconnected from the language areas of the left hemisphere. Writing with the right hand is normal because of the intact connections of the left motor cortex and the language areas. Figure 5-5 demonstrates the normal pathways required for writing. It is apparent that the callosal lesion ($F_1$) interrupts the language message going to the right hemisphere.

There are also single case reports in which isolated pure agraphia has been seen as a result of superior parietal lesions.[31]

## Psychotic Language (Bizarre Language Output)

Rambling, disjointed, neologistic language can be seen in severe psychosis (especially schizophrenia), advanced organic dementia, delirium, and fluent jargon aphasia. Differentiation among these conditions on the basis of spontaneous speech alone may be difficult. Historical data are invaluable: an acute onset of gross language disturbance in the elderly favors the diagnosis of a stroke with aphasia or delirium; a prolonged history of language deterioration in the young patient favors a diagnosis of schizophrenia or an unusual organic lesion such as a left-hemisphere glioma; a gradual deterioration of language in the older patient suggests a diagnosis of dementia or a focal brain lesion such as a left-hemisphere tumor or subdural hematoma. Unfortunately, detailed historical information is often unavailable, and a tentative diagnosis must be based upon mental status findings alone.

Each of the above conditions has certain features that help to distinguish it from the others. Systematized paranoid delusions may be seen in both aphasia and dementia. However, such delusions are more common in schizophrenia. Neologisms produced by schizophrenic patients tend to be infrequent in number, but when present, are usually consistent and symbolic (e.g., one paranoid schizophrenic patient repeatedly referred to the "frinky-franks" that were placed in the walls to watch him). Neologisms produced by aphasic patients tend to be random, very frequent, and nonsymbolic (e.g., "The walret is the you know, wimbit, lep, olla other one"). Demented patients will frequently have word-finding difficulty and will produce circumlocutory speech with some paraphasias. Their speech is generally more comprehensible, however, and less paraphasic than that of the patient with aphasia.

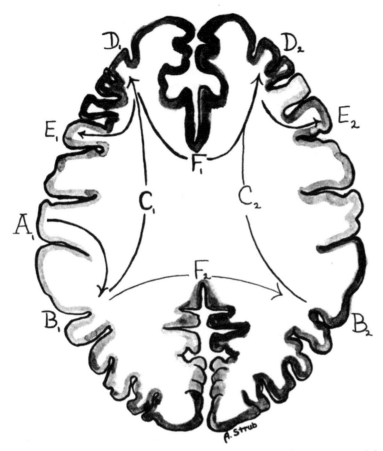

FIGURE 5-5. The written message originates in the posterior language area of the dominant hemisphere ($B_1$). The message is transferred via the arcuate fasciculus ($C_1$) to the premotor area in the same hemisphere ($D_1$). Motor patterns are transferred to the motor strip ($E_1$) for innervation of the right hand. The message must cross via the anterior corpus callosum ($F_1$) to the right motor system ($D_2$, $E_2$) for innervation of the left hand. The pathway $F_2$ is not a significant pathway for transferring the written message to the right motor area.

Because it is difficult to differentiate among these conditions by listening to spontaneous speech alone, complete language testing is essential. Careful comprehension testing reveals that jargon aphasic patients are unable to understand even very simple commands. Demented, delirious, or schizophrenic patients will have adequate comprehension, but they may be difficult to evaluate because of a lack of cooperation. Testing repetition will usually demonstrate inferior performance by aphasic patients. Naming tasks will clearly reveal aphasic patients' language problems by their production of paraphasic errors. The aphasic patient who is shown a key may say "Pel, klo, klep, kleep . . . key"; whereas the schizophrenic patient may call it a "key sort of watching tower thing." In this instance, the schizophrenic patient correctly identified the object, but incorporated it into his disordered thought process. Delirious or demented patients usually will have some naming trouble, but not as severe as that seen in aphasic patients nor as bizarre as that seen in schizophrenic patients. When asked to name a key, the demented patient might well answer, "lock, no . . . the lock keyer . . . key!"

The differential diagnosis of these conditions is important because a misdiagnosis may lead to gross mismanagement. For example, a very robust 80-year-old retired grocer began answering questions inappropriately at dinner one evening. Becoming concerned, his wife continued to ask questions, which the husband was unable to answer appropriately. He became frustrated, angry, and agitated. The wife became frightened and called the police. Because of his aggressive behavior, the man was jailed for 3 days. He was then transferred to a psychiatric hospital, where he remained for an additional 3 days before a neurologist diagnosed a Wernicke's aphasia secondary to a middle cerebral artery thrombosis. Mistakes such as this can be made unless a careful mental status examination is performed.

Differentiating the demented from the schizophrenic patient is a more difficult task. On complete examination, the demented patient may show problems with praxis and drawing that help in making the clinical diagnosis. The demented patient may show distinct organic patterns of errors on drawings (see Chapter 7). The schizophrenic patient often distorts drawings, but usually can make recognizable copies of designs and figures. Ideational apraxia (see Chapter 9), which is demonstrated by asking the patient to fold a letter and place it in an envelope, is often present in the demented patient but not in the schizophrenic patient. Some clues to the differential diagnosis may be obtained from the bedside mental status examination; however, a complete neuropsychological evaluation and other neurodiagnostic tests are often needed to make a final diagnosis.

## Nonorganic Speech and Language Disorders

These are several types of functional speech disorders that can be mistaken for organic language patterns. Some neurotic patients will convert anxiety into a halting, effortful, telegraphic speech pattern (e.g., "Me want go home see wife"). These patients have normal comprehension, repetition, and naming, but reduced verbal fluency. Reading and writing are also intact, but are carried out in the same slow, effortful fashion. Mild dysarthria may also be present. These patients may require the help of both psychiatrists and speech pathologists to alter their speech patterns.

Other functional patients develop and acute aphonia (total inability to adduct the vocal cords and make audible sounds). Aphonia may arise as a pure conversion symptom or, more commonly, as a sequela to an insult to the speech apparatus. One middle-aged patient remained aphonic for 2 months after awakening from surgery with an endotracheal tube in place. Aphonic patients breathe normally and show no evidence of stridor. They communicate well by gesture, mouthing words, and writing. This type of functional overlay is well known to speech pathologists and responds well to therapy.

Elective mutism is another functional speech disorder that may be seen in either children or emotionally disturbed adults. It is characterized by a willful reluctance or an outright refusal to speak. The disorder may be complete (i.e., an absolute lack of speech in all situations) or relative (i.e., selective communication with a small circle of intimates). The speech, when present, may be limited to a mouthing of words, whispering, or a slow, labored, halting production. The electively mute adult typically has no language deficit and is physiologically capable of producing speech sounds. Some patients, especially children, do have a basic organic language disorder with considerable emotional overlay. The mutism is often resistant to the usual forms of speech therapy and psychotherapy,[27] but it does respond to behavior modification.[26]

## SUMMARY

Language is a very complex and interesting higher-cognitive function. Because of the unique relationship of language and cerebral dominance, most acquired language disorders are pathognomonic of left-hemisphere damage. Careful evaluation of language functions can localize the lesion within the dominant hemisphere. Language is of critical importance for many other cognitive functions; thus, the subsequent parts of the mental status examination must be administered and interpreted with some caution in aphasic patients.

## REFERENCES

1. Albert, M. L.: Language in normal and dementing elderly. In Obler, L. V. and Albert, M. L. (eds.): Language and Communication in the Elderly. Lexington Books, Lexington, Mass., 1980, pp. 145–150.

2. Albert, M. L., et al: Clinical Aspects of Dysphasia. Springer-Verlag, Vienna, 1981.
3. Benson, D. F.: Fluency in aphasia: Correlation with radioactive scan localization. Cortex 3:373, 1967.
4. Benson, D. F.: Psychiatric aspects of aphasia. Br J Psychiatry 123:555, 1973.
5. Benson, D. F. and Geschwind, N.: Cerebral dominance and its disturbances. Pediatr Clin North Am 15:759, 1968.
6. Bogan, J.: Wernicke's area: Where is it? Thoughts about (and against) cortical localization. Paper presented at the 13th Annual Meeting of the Academy of Aphasia. Victoria, British Columbia, October 5, 1975.
7. Borkowski, J. G., Benton, A. L., and Spreen, O.: Word fluency and brain damage. Neuropsychologia 5:135, 1967.
8. Brown, J. W. and Hécaen, H.: Lateralization and language representation. Neurology 26:183, 1976.
9. Caramazza, A.: The logic of neuropsychological research and the problem of patient classification in aphasia. Brain Lang 21:9, 1984.
10. Cummings, J. L. and Benson, D. F.: Dementia: A Clinical Approach. Butterworth & Co, Boston, 1983.
11. Damasio, A. R., et al: Aphasia with nonhemorrhagic lesions in the basal ganglia and internal capsule. Arch Neurol 39:15, 1982.
12. Damasio, H. and Damasio, A. R.: The anatomical basis of conduction aphasia. Brain 103:337, 1980.
13. Dejerine, J.: Des differentes verietes de cecite verbale. Mem Soc Biology 1892, pp. 1–30.
14. Geschwind, N.: Disconnection syndromes in animals and man. II. Brain 88:585, 1965.
15. Geschwind, N.: Current concepts in aphasia. N Engl J Med 284:654, 1971.
16. Geschwind, N., Quadfasel, F., and Segarra, J.: Isolation of the speech area. Neuropsychologia 6:327, 1968.
17. Gloning, I., et al: Comparison of verbal behavior in right-handed and non–right-handed patients with anatomically verified lesions of one hemisphere. Cortex 5:43, 1969.
18. Gloning, K.: Handedness and aphasia. Neuropsychologia 15:355, 1977.
19. Goodglass, H. and Kaplan, E.: The Assessment of Aphasia and Related Disorders, ed. 2. Lea & Febiger, Philadelphia, 1983.
20. Hécaen, H. and de Ajuriaguerra, J.: Left Handedness: Manual Superiority and Cerebral Dominance. Grune & Stratton, New York, 1964.
21. Luria, A. R.: On quasi-aphasia speech disturbances in lesions of the deep structures of the brain. Brain Lang 4:432, 1977.
22. Metter, E. J., et al: Comparison of metabolic rates, language and memory in subcortical aphasias. Brain Lang 19:33, 1983.
23. Mohr, J. P.: Broca's area and Broca's aphasia. In Whitaker, H. and Whitaker, H. (eds.): Studies in Neurolinguistics (Perspectives in Neurolinguistics and Psycholinguistics, Vol. 1). Academic Press, New York, 1976, pp. 201–235.
24. Mohr, J. P., Watters, W. C., and Duncan, A. W.: Thalamic hemorrhage and aphasia. Brain Lang 2:3, 1975.
25. Naeser, M. A., et al: Aphasia with predominantly subcortical lesion sites: Description of three capsular/putaminal aphasia syndromes. Arch Neurol 39:2, 1982.
26. Norman, A. and Broman, H.: Volume feedback and generalization techniques in shaping speech of an electively mute boy: A case study. Percept Mot Skills 31:463, 1970.
27. Reed, G.: Elective mutism in children: A re-appraisal. J Child Psychol Psychiatry 4:99, 1963.

28. Rubens, A. B. and Kertesz, A.: The localization of lesions in transcortical aphasias. In Kertesz, A. (ed.): Localization in Neuropsychology. Academic Press, New York, 1983, pp. 245–268.
29. Strub, R. L.: Mental disorders in brain disease. In Vinken, P. J., Bruyn, G. W., and Klawans, H. L. (eds.): Handbook of Clinical Neurology, Vol. 46, Neurobehavioral Disorders. (in press)
30. Vargo, M. E. and Black, F. W.: Normative data for the Spreen-Benton Sentence Repetition Test. Cortex (in press)
31. Vignolo, L. A.: Modality specific disorders of written language. In Kertesz, A. (ed.): Localization in Neuropsychology. Academic Press, New York, 1983, pp. 357–369.
32. Wada, J.: A new method for the determination of the side of cerebral speech dominance: A preliminary report on the intracarotid injection of sodium amytal in man. Med Biol 14:221, 1949.
33. Wilson, R. S., Kaszniak, A. W., and Fox, J. H.: Remote memory in senile dementia. Cortex 17:41, 1981.
34. Zangwill, O. L.: Two cases of crossed aphasia in dextrals. Neuropsychologia 17:167, 1979.

# CHAPTER 6

# Memory

Disturbances in memory are the most common initial complaint—and often the most disabling feature—of early organic brain disease. Almost all patients with dementia show early memory problems such as losing track of the date, forgetting work details, or failing to remember commitments that fall outside of their daily routines. This problem is insidious and makes it impossible for the patient to function effectively. There can be devastating effects on social and vocational adjustment before the organic nature of the problem is fully appreciated. Recognition of this memory difficulty allows the clinician and the family to help the patient avoid potential personal catastrophe. Careful attention to memory testing can often demonstrate the presence of an organic disorder even before abnormal findings are noted on standard neurologic examination.

Various organic diseases result in different types of memory disturbance (e.g., severe memory deficit in relative isolation in Korsakoff's syndrome, memory difficulty compounded by inattention and agitation in the confusional states, or impaired memory associated with general cognitive dysfunction in dementia). In each of these diseases, memory is disturbed by different pathophysiologic mechanisms.

Not all memory difficulties are organic in origin. Depressed and anxious patients, as well as other patients with significant psychiatric disease, often have apparent difficulty with memory. Since performance on memory testing requires maximum patient cooperation and effort, the emotionally disturbed patient will often perform poorly. The misdiagnosis of depression as dementia or the reverse is a serious diagnostic error that can lead to months or even years of inappropriate treatment. This can be a difficult differential diagnostic problem. However, full neurologic, psychiatric, and psychologic evaluation can almost always lead to the appropriate diagnosis.

# TERMINOLOGY

Memory is a general term for a mental process that allows the individual to store experiences and perceptions for recall at a later time. The time span for recall can be as short as a few seconds, as in a digit repetition task, or as long as many years, as in the recall of childhood experiences. The memory process consists of several stages. In the first, the information is received and registered by a particular sensory modality (e.g., touch, auditory, or visual). Once the sensory input has been received and registered, that information is held temporarily in short-term memory. The second step consists of storing or retaining the information in a more permanent form (long-term memory). This storage process is enhanced by repetition or by association with other information that is already in storage.[19] Storage is an active process that requires effort through practice and rehearsal.[17] The final step in the memory process is the recall or retrieval of the stored information. The retrieval step is an active process of mobilizing stored information. Each stage in the total memory process relies upon the integrity of the previous steps. Any interruption in the hierarchy may prevent the storage or retrieval of a memory. Memory studies have demonstrated that certain aspects of memory have distinct neuroanatomic substrates and are subject to specific disease processes.

Clinically, memory is subdivided into three basic types based upon the time span between stimulus presentation and memory retrieval. The terms "immediate," "recent," and "remote" are commonly used to denote these basic types. Unfortunately, these terms are descriptive, and the time span implied is not well defined in clinical use. Immediate memory or immediate recall refers to the recall of a memory trace after an interval of a few seconds, as in repetition of a series of digits. The term short-term memory is also used by some to describe the same task.

Recent memory is a term that refers to the patient's capacity to remember day-to-day events (e.g., the date, the doctor's name, what he or she ate for breakfast, or recent news events). More strictly defined, recent memory is the ability to learn new material and to retrieve that material after an interval of minutes, hours, or days.

Remote memory is traditionally used to refer to the recollection of very early events, such as the names of teachers and old school friends, birth dates, and historical facts. In patients with a specific defect in new learning (recent memory), remote memory refers to the recall of events that occurred prior to the onset of the recent memory defect.

Amnesia is a general term for a defect in memory. Although the term may be applied to a broad spectrum of memory defects, it is most commonly used to label patients with severe and relatively isolated memory deficits (e.g., Korsakoff's syndrome or post-traumatic amnesia). The inability to learn new material is called anterograde amnesia. Retrograde amnesia refers to amnesia for events that occurred prior to a brain insult. The time period may be as short as a few seconds or as long as several years. It is most commonly seen with head trauma, but may also follow any major brain insult (e.g., stroke). The term amnesia is also used to refer to psychogenic amnesia, in which the patient blocks out a period of time. These patients do not demonstrate a recent memory deficit or an inability to learn on specific memory testing.

## EVALUATION

In the thorough mental status examination, the various aspects of memory should be assessed in some detail. This will allow the examiner to distinguish the type of memory deficit (if any), the degree of memory loss, and the impact of the memory deficit upon the patient's ability to function in a vocational or social role.

The patient will commonly show different performance levels on various memory tests, depending upon the nature of the disorder (e.g., the patient with Korsakoff's syndrome will be able to respond very adequately to questions regarding more remote events, but will be unable to learn new material). The use of several different memory tests is also of clinical importance. Brain-damaged patients will demonstrate differences in the incidence, nature, and degree of memory deficits based upon the type of test utilized and the nature and location of their lesions.[2,3,8,13]

The accurate assessment of memory requires that any question asked by the examiner be verifiable from a source other than the patient. For example, it does very little good to ask patients when they graduated from high school or what they ate for lunch if the examiner is unable to ascertain the accuracy of the patients' responses. Many patients with readily demonstrable memory deficits will deny their problem and will produce confabulated answers. Such responses may appear perfectly appropriate to the naive examiner who is unable to verify their accuracy. Personal information concerning the patient's social history, lifestyle, vocation, and so forth may be verified by the doctor if he or she has followed the patient for some time. In other cases, the patient's family can verify this information. Material that cannot be accurately verified should not be used in the assessment of memory.

Historical facts (e.g., "When was World War II?" or "Who was the president before Mr. Reagan?") are commonly used by examiners to screen memory. The basic knowledge of such information is closely related to the patient's basic premorbid intellectual level, education, and general social exposure. These factors must be considered when using historical facts to test memory. If used at all, questions related to historical material must be tailored to the background of the individual patient, and the patient's responses must be interpreted in the context of this information.

One of the most sensitive and valid tests of memory is to require the patient to learn new material over time. The use of this technique eliminates some of the dangers of unverified material and unknown social background. New learning is an active memory process that requires more expenditure of effort on the patient's part than does the mere recall of personal or historical facts.

When evaluating memory, the examiner must be aware of a number of more basic processes that can result in impaired performance even in the patient without a true memory deficit. Performance on memory tests requires sustained attention. Accordingly, patients with attention disorders of any etiology will be unable to perform optimally on such tests. Similarly, the patient in an acute confusional state or with a severe psychogenic disturbance will have impaired attention, which will hinder memory performance. Disturbances of basic sensory, motor, or language functions that interfere with comprehension or expression will result in impaired memory test performance. Poor memory performance by deaf, aphasic, acutely confused, psychotic, or grossly inattentive patients reflects defects in these more basic processes and should not be misinterpreted as evidence of specific memory deficits. Valid memory testing presumes that the patient is reasonably attentive, is capable of relating to and cooperating with the examiner, and has no defect that impairs the comprehension or expression of language.

Because of the clinical and social importance of memory, we have selected a number of memory tests that enable the examiner to assess a variety of memory processes.

## Immediate Recall (Short-Term Memory)

Immediate recall is usually tested by digit repetition. This is covered in detail in Chapter 4 and will not be repeated here. Although backward digit repetition has been used by some examiners to assess verbal memory, this is a highly complex task that requires several neuropsychological processes in addition to memory.[4] It is useful as a general screening test for brain dysfunction but should not be considered a test of short-term memory in isolation.

# Orientation

The patient's ability to orient himself or herself with respect to person (who he or she is), time (the date, and so forth), and place (where he or she is) is important preliminary information and should be evaluated early in the examination of memory functioning.

Orientation to place and time are actually measures of recent memory since they test the patient's ability to learn these continuing changes. If a patient is not fully oriented, this alone suggests a significant recent memory deficit.

*Directions.* The patient should be asked the following questions in sequence. Questions may be paraphrased when necessary to ensure clarity. If the patient fails these items, tell the patient the correct answers and have him or her repeat them, and then have the patient recall the answers several minutes later. Failure at this level verifies very poor learning ability and will predict deficient performance on subsequent memory tasks.

1. Person
   a. Name      What is your name?
   b. Age      How old are you?
   c. Birthdate      When is your birthday?
        (day, month, year)
2. Place
   a. Location      Where are we right now?
        What is the name of this place?
        What kind of place are we in now?
   b. City location      What city are we in now?
   c. Address      What is your home address?
3. Time
   a. Date      What is today's date?
        (year, month, date)
   b. Day of the week      What day of the week is it?
   c. Time of day      What time is it right now?
   d. Season of the year      What season is it now?
   e. Time duration      How long have you been in the hospital?
        How long have we been talking?

Normal people perform perfectly on this test ($\bar{x}$ = 10.6), although somewhat less adequate scores are noted on time orientation by hospitalized patients.[22] More than two errors is indicative of impaired orientation.

## Remote Memory

Tests in this section evaluate the patient's ability to recall events of both a personal and historical nature. As emphasized, personal events must be verifiable by a reliable source other than the patient; the performance on the recall of historical information must be interpreted in the light of the patient's premorbid intelligence, education, and social experience.

  1. Personal information
    a. Where were you born?
    b. School information:    Where did you go to school?
                                When did you attend school?
                                Where is your school located?
    c. Vocational history:    What do you do for work?
                                Where have you worked?
                                When did you work at those places?
    d. Family information:    What is your wife's (children's) name?
                                  How old is your wife (children)?
                                What was your mother's maiden name?

Personal information items are completed with approximately equal accuracy by both normal patients and patients with mild, nonspecific brain damage. While impaired performance is pathologic, this test does not efficiently differentiate between groups.[22]

  2. Historical facts
    a. Ask the patient to name four people who have been president during the patient's lifetime. The normal patient should be able to accomplish this task without difficulty.
    b. Ask the patient to name the last war in which the United States was directly involved. At the time of this writing, the correct response would be the war in Vietnam. An older patient may name either the Korean War or World War II. If the patient gives either response, ask him or her about any recollection of the Vietnam war. If the patient has no memory for this major event, this implies deficient memory.

## New-Learning Ability

This section assesses the patient's ability to actively learn new material (to lay down new memories). Adequate performance requires the integrity of the total memory system: recognition and registration of the initial sensory input, retention and storage of the information, and recall or retrieval of the stored information. An interruption in any of these stages will impair new-learning ability. A careful clinical examination of how the patient fails a particular task may often provide valuable information as to the nature of the impaired process.

Four Unrelated Words

*Directions.* Tell the patient, "I am going to tell you four words that I would like you to remember. In a few minutes, I will ask you to recall these words." To ensure that the patient has heard, understood, and initially retained the four words, have him or her repeat the words after their presentation. Correct any errors made on immediate repetition. To eliminate possible mental rehearsal, interference should be used between presentation and recall of the words. Accordingly, the examiner may wish to present the four words prior to the remote memory examination. After 5 minutes, ask for the recall of the four words. Information concerning the duration of memory can be obtained by asking for a recall of the words after 10 and 30 minutes. The following words have been selected because of their semantic and phonemic diversity.

*Test Items*

| 1. Brown | 1. Fun |
| 2. Honesty | 2. Carrot |
| 3. Tulip | 3. Ankle |
| 4. Eyedropper | 4. Loyalty |

*Scoring.* The normal patient is expected to accurately recall the four words after a 10-minute delay. After a 30-minute delay, at least three ($\bar{x} = 3.6$) of the four words should be recalled. Performance of less than three words recalled at either 10 or 30 minutes is indicative of impaired new-learning ability.[22] When a patient is unable to recall a word, it is often possible to obtain an indication of memory storage by the use of verbal cues. Semantic cues relating to the category of the named object (e.g., "one word was a color"), phonemic cues utilizing syllabic components of the word (e.g., "Hon ... hones ... honest ... honesty"), and contextual cues (e.g., "A common flower in Holland is a _____") may be used. If a patient is unable to either spontaneously recall the words or to recall them with cues, the examiner may resort to asking the patient if he or she recognizes the appropriate word from a series of words (e.g., "Was the color red, green, brown, or yellow?").

Verbal Story for Immediate Recall

*Directions.* Tell the patient, "I am going to read you a short paragraph. Listen carefully, because when I finish reading, I want you to tell me everything that I told you." After reading the story, say, "Now tell me everything that you can remember of the story. Start at the beginning of the story and tell me all that happened." The separate items in the story are indicated by slash (/) marks. As the patient retells the story, indicate the number of ideas recalled. In patients with good immediate recall, it may be useful to ask for another recall after 30 minutes. This is a sensitive method of assessing short-term verbal recall.

### Test Item

It was July / and the Rogers / had packed up / their four children / in the station wagon / and were off / on vacation.

They were taking / their yearly trip / to the beach / at Gulf Shores. / This year / they were making / a special / 2-day stop / at the World's Fair / in New Orleans.

After a long day's drive / they arrived / at the motel / only to discover / that in their excitement / they had left / the twins / and their suitcases / in the front yard.

*Scoring.* The story contains 26 relatively separate ideas, or information items. In our experience, the average patient should be expected to produce at least eight of these items on immediate recall. Less adequate performance by the nonretarded patient indicates defective verbal recall ability. The story included in the first edition of this book significantly discriminated between brain-damaged and low-IQ normal groups. The present story has not yet been normed.

Visual Memory (Hidden Objects)

*Directions.* Visual memory testing should be used with all patients, but it is especially useful in evaluating the memory of aphasic patients. The examiner may utilize any four or five small, easily recognizable objects that may be readily hidden in the patient's vicinity. We have commonly used items such as a pen, a watch, keys, coins, and eyeglasses. The use of four or five items provides a reasonable span for most patients. The objects are hidden while the patient is watching. Name each item as it is hidden to ensure that the patient is aware of what object was hidden in what place. After hiding the objects, the examiner should provide interfering stimuli by administering another mental status task, asking the patient routine questions, or engaging the patient in general conversation. An interference period of 10 minutes should suffice. After this period, ask the patient to find each of the hidden objects. If the patient is unable to recall the location of any object, ask him or her to name the hidden object.

*Scoring.* The average patient should find each hidden object after a 10-minute delay without difficulty. Less adequate performance (fewer than 3 objects) indicates impaired visual memory. A patient with aphasia should be able to find the objects, but may not be able to name them.

## Visual Memory (Visual Design Reproduction)

This is a part of most memory batteries. It is a very useful test item, but can be considered optional when used as a component of the mental status examination. It is not a test of visual memory alone, since problems with constructional ability (see Chapter 7) will also adversely affect performance.

*Directions.* The following subtest utilizes four simple line drawings of increasing complexity. We recommend that the examiner provide standardized stimuli cards to ensure uniformity, although the examiner may choose to draw each design at the bedside. The patient is required to reproduce each of the four designs on a piece of white paper after a 5-second presentation of the design and a 10-second delay before beginning. The following instructions are given: "I am now going to show you some simple drawings. I want you to look at each drawing as I show it to you. Be sure to look at it carefully so that you can draw what you have seen from memory. Do not draw the design until I have told you to begin." (Fig. 6-1)

*Scoring.* Each design may be scored on a four-point scale with values from 0 to 3. The higher the score, the more adequate the reproduction. The following scoring system may be used to aid the examiner in quantifying performance on this test:

| | |
|---|---|
| 0—Poor | Given for a failure to recall and reproduce the design. |
| 1—Fair | Given for recognizable but distorted, rotated, partially omitted, or confabulated features of the design. |
| 2—Good | Given for easily recognizable designs with minor errors of integration, omission, or addition. |
| 3—Excellent | Given for perfect (or near perfect) reproductions of the items with all appropriate components, placements, and integration. |

Representative clinical examples of poor, fair, good, and excellent drawings are shown in Figures 6-2 through 6-5 to aid the examiner in rating each design.

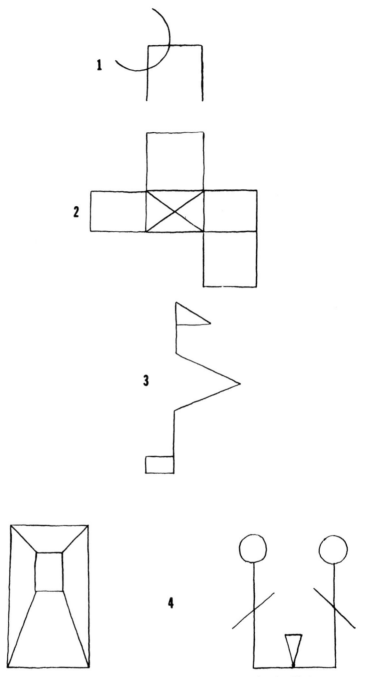

FIGURE 6-1. Test items for Visual Design Reproduction Test.

FIGURE 6-2. Renderings of design 1, with scores of 0 (poor) through 3 (excellent).

0

1

2

3

FIGURE 6-3. Renderings of design 2, with scores of 0 (poor) through 3 (excellent).

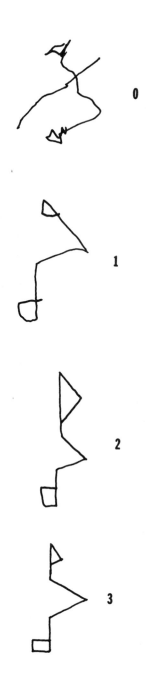

0

1

2

3

FIGURE 6-4. Renderings of design 3, with scores of 0 (poor) through 3 (excellent).

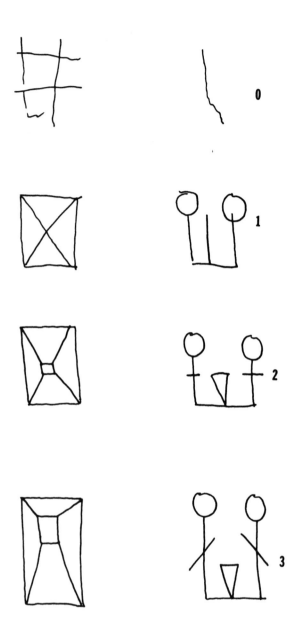

FIGURE 6-5. Renderings of design 4, with scores of 0 (poor) through 3 (excellent).

The average patient should produce reproductions of each design at the 2 and 3 scoring levels. All designs should be recalled. Less adequate performance indicates a deficit in visual memory.

Paired Associate Learning (PAL)

This test is commonly used in standard memory batteries and is another good and highly sensitive measure of new-learning ability.

*Directions.* Tell the patient, "I am going to read you a list of words, two at a time. Listen carefully because I will expect you to remember the words that go together. For example, if the words were big—little, I would expect you to say the word little after I said the word big." When the patient is clear as to the directions, continue as follows: "Now listen carefully to the words as I read them." Read the first presentation at the rate of one pair every 2 seconds. After reading the first presentation, test for recall by presenting the first recall list. Give the first word of a pair and allow 5 seconds for a response. If the patient gives a correct response, say "That's right" and proceed with the next pair. If the patient gives an incorrect response, say "No," provide the correct word, and proceed to the next pair.

After the first recall has been completed, allow a 10-second interval and give the second presentation list, proceeding as before.

*Test Items*

### Presentation Lists

| *First Presentation* | *Second Presentation* |
|---|---|
| Weather—Bag | House—Income |
| High—Low | Weather—Bag |
| House—Income | Book—Page |
| Book—Page | High—Low |

### Recall Lists

| *First Recall* | *Second Recall* |
|---|---|
| House—_____ | High—_____ |
| High—_____ | House—_____ |
| Weather—_____ | Book—_____ |
| Book—_____ | Weather—_____ |

*Scoring.* The normal patient is expected to recall the two "easy" paired associates (high—low, book—page) and at least one of the "hard" associates on the first recall trial, and to recall all paired associates on the second trial. Less adequate performance is indicative of impaired new-learning ability.[22] Some patients will be able to learn the paired

TABLE 6-1. Statistical Comparison of Memory Tests

| Variable | Brain Damaged Mean | Low-IQ Normal Mean | F |
|---|---|---|---|
| Total Score | 33.4 | 50 | 28.0[‡] |
| Digit Repetition | 4.2 | 4.8 | 1.9 |
| Vigilance errors | 10.2 | 0.2 | 5.5[†] |
| Orientation | 8.7 | 10.6 | 13.3[‡] |
| Person | 2.6 | 3.0 | 7.5[‡] |
| Place | 2.7 | 3.0 | 3.4[*] |
| Time | 3.4 | 4.6 | 8.4[‡] |
| Remote Memory | | | |
| Personal Information | 3.4 | 3.9 | 3.1 |
| Historical Facts | 1.3 | 1.5 | 3.2 |
| Four Words — 10 minutes | 1.9 | 3.6 | 15.1[‡] |
| Four Words — 30 minutes | 1.8 | 3.9 | 20.4[‡] |
| Visual Memory | | | |
| Hidden objects found (4) | 1.3 | 3.7 | 10.8[‡] |
| Hidden objects named | 1.0 | 0.2 | 3.1 |
| Paired Associate Learning | | | |
| Easy | 2.1 | 3.0 | 12.6[‡] |
| Difficult | 1.4 | 3.0 | 9.7[‡] |
| Total | 3.5 | 6.0 | 15.6[‡] |

* $p > 0.05$
† $p > 0.01$
‡ $p > 0.001$

words with strong natural associations but will be unable to learn the pairs without such associations. This discrepancy demonstrates a reliance upon semantic cues and an inability to learn new material that cannot be associated with memories already in storage. The total PAL score is the best measure of verbal learning.

The results of a statistical comparison of these memory tests between groups with mixed brain damage and normal patients with IQs below 80 appear in Table 6-1. Differences in age and education were controlled.[22]

## CLINICAL IMPLICATIONS

Some aspects of the memory process can be associated with certain neuroanatomic structures or neuronal systems. Pathologic studies have amply documented that limbic structures are involved in the long-term storage and retrieval of recent information.[6,16,20,28] However, the structures that are required for immediate recall and remote memory are not as well established. Although all memory traces—visual, verbal, and tactile—are most likely stored in the neocortex, there are many subcortical structures that are necessary for the total memory process (registration, storage, and retrieval). Damage or disruption of cortical or subcortical systems will result in different patterns of dysfunction. Accordingly, the anatomy of memory is discussed in a way that allows the correlation of specific structure, memory type, and clinical condition.

## Immediate Recall

The immediate recall of digits is a process that does not require any long-term storage of information, but it does require initial registration, short-term holding, and verbal repetition. This entire process can be performed by the language cortex surrounding the sylvian fissure. This has been demonstrated in patients with transcortical aphasia.[11] The exact mechanism by which these short-term memories are maintained within the language system is not known. Reverberating circuits may be established, or patterns of cortical after-image may be present. Whatever change does occur, it is not long lasting. Efficient short-term memory is not a passive process. A digit sequence task will be performed much better if active mental rehearsal takes place. Digits are typically presented at 1-second intervals, but each digit takes approximately 200 milliseconds to present. The 800 milliseconds between digits allows ample time for rehearsal and, thus, increased efficiency in repetition. If the patient actively groups digits into two- or three-digit sets, his or her performance will improve. A third and always very important element in all memory processing is the association of the new material with previously stored information. A digit sequence that is similar to an old phone number or address will be much more easily recalled than a completely unique random sequence. Short-term memory (immediate recall) is a distinct property of the cortical sensory, motor, and integrative areas necessary to register, recall, and produce the original stimulus. It does not require the limbic systems necessary for long-term storage and permanent memory formation.

If there is any damage to or disruption of these basic sensory or motor areas, then short-term memory will be faulty. In digit repetition, the language system is essential; therefore, any degree of aphasia (excluding the transcortical aphasias) can cause disruption of immediate memory functioning. This repetition failure is particularly pronounced in conduction aphasia.[27] The primary deficit in conduction aphasia is an inability to repeat. Whether this repetition failure is a defect in language or short-term memory is an open question that may, in fact, reflect an argument of semantics.

Probably the most common cause of failure on short-term memory tasks is inattention.[23] If a patient's attention strays from the stimulus during presentation, the information will be imperfectly registered. Similarly, if the patient is inattentive during the repetition phase and time pauses occur, the memory trace will fade. Inattention can be organic, as in confusional states and dementia, or functional, as in anxiety and depression. The clinical implications of these attentional disturbances are discussed fully in Chapters 3 and 4.

The demented patient will have difficulty with immediate memory for several reasons: such patients are often inattentive; they have cortical atrophy, which affects their basic language and other sensory-motor integration systems; and they have general intellectual deterioration.[30]

## Recent Memory

In general, the ability to store and then retrieve new material (recent memory, new learning, or memorizing) presumes intact registration, retention, and short-term storage. If the material is familiar and can be associated with information in long-term storage, the process is easier and relies less on short-term storage.[19]

Certain limbic structures are required to ensure storage and retrieval. The hippocampi, the mamillary bodies, and the dorsal medial nuclei of the thalami are essential subcortical links in the storage and retrieval of both verbal and nonverbal memories.[6,20,28] Actual memories are probably not stored in these structures, but the limbic system seems to act as the mechanism to store and retrieve memories from the cortex.

Whenever these subcortical structures are destroyed or severely damaged, the patient is rendered unable to learn new material (anterograde amnesia) or to retrieve memories from the recent past (retrograde amnesia). These patients literally become fixed in time and are unable to record the passing of events from that time onward. There are certain clinical situations in which these limbic structures are damaged in isolation. Such patients develop a profound organic amnesic state. This condition is characterized clinically by the following findings: (1) severe anterograde amnesia; (2) moderate to severe retrograde amnesia, which can extend back for several years; and, usually, (3) confabulation during the acute stage. In the face of this devastating memory impairment, the patients have remarkably intact immediate memory as assessed by digit repetition and other short-term memory tests. These patients also demonstrate no change in premorbid levels of intelligence. They carry on coherent, intelligent conversations that appear abnormal only when recent events are discussed. Because the patients do not remember the date, place, and recent events, they appear confused. This confusion, which is due to their memory problems, can be easily misinterpreted as the classic acute confusional state described in Chapter 2. Careful observation and testing will prevent this diagnostic error.

This dramatic organic amnesic state has been seen secondary to bilateral temporal lobectomy, herpes simplex encephalitis, and bilateral hippocampal infarction. In these cases, the hippocampus has been completely destroyed bilaterally. A similar memory deficit is seen clinically in Korsakoff's syndrome (a syndrome of thiamine depletion seen in chronic alcoholism and severe malnutrition). In Korsakoff's syndrome, the lesions involve bilateral destruction of the mamillary bodies and the dorsal medial nuclei of the thalami. The patient with Korsakoff's syndrome frequently, but not invariably, goes through an acute encephalopathy (Wernicke's encephalopathy) at the onset of the memory difficulty. Vascular or traumatic lesions of the dorsal medial thalamus also cause severe organic amnesia.[24,26]

In Alzheimer's dementia, patients also have defects in new learning. These defects are due in part to a gradual degeneration of the cells in the hippocampus. The memory loss in the atrophic dementias is complex, however, and will be discussed more fully in the section that deals with remote memory.

The most familiar amnesia to the layperson is the memory loss that occurs after head injury. Patients with acute head injury almost always have some degree of retrograde amnesia for the time immediately preceding the injury, and they usually have transient difficulty learning new material after the trauma. In head trauma, the temporal lobes are commonly concussed against the bony confines of the middle fossa. This trauma causes a physiologic disruption of hippocampal function, which in turn disturbs memory storage and retrieval. Post-traumatic amnesia is usually reversible; but in cases of significant temporal lobe damage, the memory loss can be permanent. Repeated concussion such as that seen in boxers may result in gradual, but permanent, memory disturbance. An interesting feature of the amnesia seen with acute head injury is that the retrograde amnesic period will shorten in the days following recovery of consciousness. Initially, the patient may not recall events that occurred years preceding the accident. Within several days, the patient may remember all but the few minutes that immediately preceded the accident. This shrinking retrograde amnesia verifies that the injury did not eliminate the memories from storage, but merely rendered them temporarily irretrievable.[1,14]

Clinically, the memory disturbance in the various types of organic amnesias is similar (i.e., the patients cannot recall recent information). On experimental tasks, however, it has been shown that patients with Korsakoff's syndrome, whose damage is in the thalamus and mamillary body, have actually retained a considerable amount of the material presented to them, but are unaware of this. The deficit is with retrieving and realizing that the information has been presented rather than with the storage process. Patients with hippocampal and temporal lobe damage have both a storage and a retrieval defect. As mentioned above, the fact that the cortex of the Korsakoff patient has stored the engrams for the memory does not help the patient clinically, since he or she does not realize that they are stored and cannot use the information.[29]

Transient global amnesia is another type of organic memory problem. This syndrome probably involves transient ischemia of both medial temporal lobes secondary to decreased perfusion in the territory of the posterior cerebral arteries.[12,15] This syndrome is characterized by an acute, but temporary, confusional state with amnesia. The patients are disoriented to time and place and have a significant defect in new-learning ability. Recovery generally occurs within hours or days, and the patient is left with a permanent amnesia only for the duration of the episode itself. Fortunately, most episodes of transient global amnesia are temporary, although permanent memory loss has been seen in patients suffering bilateral hippocampal infarction.[7] The following case illustrates some of the essential features of this syndrome:

Dr. J. L. was a robust 68-year-old educator who was addressing a teacher's convention. In the middle of his speech, he stopped suddenly, became dazed, and began to ask where he was. He repeatedly asked, "What am I doing and where am I?" On initial neurologic examination, he was distraught and very confused. He was unable to attend well and was unable to learn new material. He did not remember arriving in New Orleans, but he did know that he was scheduled to attend the convention. One day later, his mental function was essentially normal except that he was amnesic for the day prior to and the day of his amnesic episode.

All of the conditions discussed thus far have resulted from bilateral lesions localized in limbic structures. Although it is true that a bilateral lesion is necessary to produce a profound memory loss, there is some loss of specific memory functions following a unilateral lesion. Unilateral dominant temporal lobectomy patients show a relative decrease in verbal learning; whereas patients with unilateral nondominant temporal lobectomies demonstrate a decrease in visual memory.[16] This pattern of differential deficits is also seen with unilateral subcortical lesions.[25]

There are various factors other than specific limbic damage that can interfere with the storage and retrieval of new material; some of these have been discussed in the previous section, but they merit additional mention here. Inattention will prevent any patient from accurately storing new material. Efficient memory storage requires close attention to the information for short-term registration and continued attention and rehearsal for storage. For this reason, new learning cannot be validly tested in inattentive patients. Aphasic patients are also at a tremendous disadvantage in any verbal learning task; if they cannot accurately comprehend or repeat verbal material, it is not valid to judge their memory capacity using that material. Nonverbal memory tasks are necessary to validly assess memory in aphasic patients. Memory test performance and intelligence are directly related; accordingly, patients' premorbid intellectual levels must be considered when interpreting the results of memory testing. Deficits in basic sensory capacity (i.e., hearing and vision) are sometimes overlooked in testing, but obviously sensory systems must be adequate for memory testing in each specific modality.

The patient's emotional state can also significantly affect new-learning ability. Very anxious patients will make errors due to inattention and distractibility. Depressed patients perform poorly on memory testing because of their inability to put forth the required effort to memorize the presented material.

Depressed patients also tend to remember negative or sad information more effectively than positive or happy events or ideas.[5] In significant depression, the decrease in motivation and learning probably involves more than pure psychological mechanisms. The underlying chemical disorder postulated in major depressive illness undoubtedly adversely affects neuronal functioning at various levels.[9]

Poor performance on memory tests is probably the single most important factor resulting in the misdiagnosis of depression as dementia.[18] Accordingly, in the patient with psychomotor retardation and memory problems, the diagnosis of depression must be considered and pursued in the evaluation process.

## Remote Memory

When a memory has remained in a person's repertoire for a number of years, it can be considered a remote, or old, memory. These memories are stored in the appropriate association cortex (e.g., language cortex for verbal material). In contrast to recent memory, remote memory does not require the limbic system for retrieval from storage. Patients with Korsakoff's syndrome or bilateral temporal lobectomy can accurately discuss personal and historical events that occurred years previously (remote memory), yet they are unable to remember what they had for breakfast that morning (recent memory).[21] There is apparently a mechanism, thus far unexplained, by which memories finally become sufficiently well established that they can be recalled without the aid of subcortical limbic structures. These remote memories can be lost only by damage to the cortical storage areas themselves. This loss of remote, or old, memories is seen in patients with the atrophic dementias (Alzheimer's and Pick's) or with any disease that damages extensive areas of the cortex. The memory disturbance in the demented patient is complex: such patients have difficulty with short-term memory because of atrophy in the basic sensory association cortex (e.g., language cortex for verbal memory); they are hampered in recent memory acquisition because of degeneration of cells in the hippocampal system; and they have defects in remote memory because of widespread cortical atrophy.

## Functional Memory Disturbances

Not all memory disorders are of organic origin, and knowledge of the functional disturbances of memory is important. The interference with memory performance that can occur secondary to anxiety and depression has been discussed previously. There are, however, several psychiatric conditions in which memory disturbances are central features. The first and most common is the dissociative state, now called psychogenic amnesia. This is the classic amnesia that has been popularized in the press and in movies. The patients either lose their identity completely (fugue state) or have periods of minutes, hours, or days when they carry out their normal life routine and later become aware that they remember nothing of what transpired during this period (dissociative state). During a dissociative or fugue state, the patients do not act confused, as do persons with transient global amnesia, and they are able to learn new material, unlike patients with organic amnesia. There should be no difficulty in differentiating the organic amnesic who cannot learn new material when tested from the psychogenic amnesic who has experienced a "memory lapse." Brief testing with the four unrelated words task or the paired associate words task should suffice.

There is one other curious pseudomemory disturbance: the Ganser syndrome, or the syndrome of approximate answers. These patients will routinely give approximate answers to all questions: for example, today is Tuesday (actually, it is Wednesday), the month is March (actually, it is April), or 2 and 2 are 5. Because their answers are so consistently close to the correct answer, it is obvious that they have more knowledge of the subject in question than they are indicating. Although the approximate answer is the most characteristic symptom, Ganser's original patients all had clouded consciousness, hallucinations, and somatic conversion symptoms.[10]

The syndrome was originally described in prisoners, but it is not exclusively seen in this population. The syndrome is uncommon and it is not seen in children. Its etiology is unclear; however, some patients have a schizophrenic disorder or an underlying organic mental disorder. The nature and inconsistency of their mental status findings strongly suggest a significant component of either hysteria or malingering. Most patients have some motivating reason to appear legally insane or incompetent.

On occasion, professed memory loss is a conscious and motivated symptom of malingering. It may be associated with other feigned neurologic or psychiatric symptoms, but can also be seen alone. The patients whom we have seen usually have a very specific, well-recognized reason for their malingering; in our experience, either avoiding prosecution by virtue of incompetence or gaining compensation for a minor head injury. On examination, these patients may give approximate answers or very bizarre answers. Their memory loss is usually inconsistent in that they may fail all memory testing but remember a football score from the previous weekend. They also claim patches of remote memory loss and at times claim not to remember their own name.

## SUMMARY

In general, memory is a hierarchical process in which information must first be registered in a basic sensory cortical area and then processed through the limbic system for new learning to occur. Finally, the material is permanently established in the appropriate association cortex. At this point, limbic retrieval is no longer required in the recall process. The immediate recall system is disturbed by damage to the primary sensory or motor cortex or by inattention. Learning is prevented by damage to the hippocampi or the dorsal medial thalamic nuclei. Old remote memories are resistant to limbic damage but will be lost when widespread cortical damage occurs. Careful testing of the various aspects of memory can frequently lead to both a clinical and an anatomic diagnosis.

## REFERENCES

1. Benson, D. F. and Geschwind, N.: Shrinking retrograde amnesia. J Neurol Neurosurg Psychiatry 30:539, 1967.
2. Benton, A. and Spreen, O.: Visual memory test performance in mentally deficient and brain-damaged patients. Am J Ment Defic 68:630, 1964.
3. Bisiach, E. and Faglioni, P.: Recognition of random shapes by patients with unilateral lesions as a function of complexity, association value, and delay. Cortex 10:101, 1974.
4. Black, F. W. and Strub, R. L.: Digit repetition performance in patients with focal brain damage. Cortex 14:12, 1978.

5. Breslow, R., Kocsis, J., and Belkin, B.: Contribution of the depressive perspective to memory function in depression. Am J Psychiatry 138:227, 1981.

6. DeJong, R., Itabashi, H., and Olson, J.: Memory loss due to hippocampal lesions. Arch Neurol 20:339, 1969.

7. DeJong, R.: The hippocampus and its role in memory. J Neurol Sci 19:73, 1973.

8. DeRenzi, E.: Nonverbal memory and hemispheric side of lesion. Neuropsychologia 6:181, 1968.

9. Folstein, M. F. and McHugh, P. P.: Dementia syndrome of depression. In Katzman, R., Terry, R. D., and Beck, K. L. (eds.): Alzheimer's Disease: Senile Dementia and Related Disorders (Aging, Vol. 7). Raven Press, New York, 1978, pp. 87–94.

10. Ganser, S. J. M.: A peculiar hysterical state. In Hirsch, S. R. and Shepherd, M. (eds.): Themes and Variations in European Psychiatry: An Anthology. J Wright, Bristol, 1974, pp. 67–77.

11. Geschwind, N., Quadfasel, F., and Segarra, J.: Isolation of the speech area. Neuropsychologia 6:327, 1968.

12. Heathfield, K., Croft, P., and Swash, M.: The syndrome of transient global amnesia. Brain 96:729, 1973.

13. Lewinsohn, P., et al: A comparison between frontal and nonfrontal right and left hemisphere brain-damaged patients. J Comp Physiol Psychol 81:248, 1972.

14. Logan, W. and Sherman, D. G.: Transient global amnesia. Stroke 14:1005, 1983.

15. Mathew, N. and Meyer, J.: Pathogenesis and natural history of transient global amnesia. Stroke 5:303, 1974.

16. Milner, B.: Intellectual functions of the temporal lobes. Psychol Bull 51:42, 1954.

17. Neisser, U.: Cognitive Psychology. Appleton-Century-Crofts, New York, 1967.

18. Nott, P. and Fleminger, J.: Presenile dementia: The difficulties of early diagnosis. Acta Psychiatr Scand 51:210, 1975.

19. Parkin, A. J.: Residual learning capability in organic amnesia. Cortex 18:417, 1982.

20. Scoville, W. and Milner, B.: Loss of recent memory after bilateral hippocampal lesions. J Neurol Neurosurg Psychiatry 20:11, 1957.

21. Selzer, B. and Benson, D. F.: The temporal pattern of retrograde amnesia in Korsakoff's disease. Neurology 24:527, 1974.

22. Simpson, N. and Black, F. W.: Validation of bedside mental status memory testing: A comparison of the Strub-Black mental status exam and the Wechsler memory scale in brain damaged patients. Paper presented at the 30th Annual Convention of the Southeastern Psychological Association, March 29, 1984, New Orleans, Louisiana.

23. Smith, A.: The Serial Sevens Subtraction Test. Arch Neurol 17:78, 1967.

24. Speedie, L. J. and Heilman, K. M.: Amnestic disturbances following infarction of the left dorsomedial nucleus of the thalamus. Neuropsychologia 20:597, 1982.

25. Speedie, L. J. and Heilman, K. M.: Anterograde memory deficits for visuospatial material after infarction of the right thalamus. Arch Neurol 40:183, 1983.

26. Squire, L. R. and Moore, R. Y.: Dorsal thalamic lesion in a noted case of human memory dysfunction. Ann Neurol 6:503, 1979.

27. Strub, R. and Gardner, H.: The repetition defect in conduction aphasia: Mnestic or linguistic? Brain Lang 1:241, 1975.

28. Victor, M., Adams, R., and Collins, G.: The Wernicke-Korsakoff Syndrome. FA Davis, Philadelphia, 1971.

29. Warrington, E. K. and Weiskrantz, L.: Amnesia: A disconnection syndrome. Neuropsychologia 20:233, 1982.

30. Wilson, R., et al: Primary memory and secondary memory in dementia of the Alzheimer type. J Clin Neuropsychol 5:337, 1983.

# CHAPTER 7

# Constructional Ability

Constructional tasks such as line drawings and block designs are extremely useful for detecting organic brain disease and should be included in all mental status examinations. Constructional ability (constructional praxis) can be defined as the capacity to draw or construct two- or three-dimensional figures or shapes. Copying line drawings using pencil on paper, reproducing matchstick patterns, and reconstructing block designs are all examples of routinely employed tests of constructional ability. This high-level nonverbal cognitive function is a very complex perceptual motor task that involves an integration of occipital, parietal, and frontal lobe function. Because of the extensive cortical area necessary to perform constructional tasks, early or subtle brain damage frequently disrupts performance. In some patients, the unsuccessful attempt to copy a simple line drawing can be the only objective evidence suggesting organic brain disease.

Despite their importance and proven clinical utility, constructional tasks are frequently not included in bedside or office mental status testing. This is due in part to the fact that very few patients actually complain of constructional impairment. Architects or engineers, whose professions require such abilities, might notice difficulties when drawing plans, reading blueprints, or translating plans into actual construction. Most patients, however, are quite surprised to find that they are unable to draw a clock or copy a block design when asked to do so. Since constructional tests take only a few minutes to perform and can yield very valuable data, we encourage every clinician to use them when performing routine mental status testing.

The term constructional ability, rather than the more classic term constructional praxis, will be used to discuss this general area of cognitive function. Praxis, in the strict sense, refers to the motor integration employed in the execution of complex learned movements. The reproduction of line drawings or block designs involves more than the organization of skilled hand movements. Such reproduction requires accurate visual perception, integration of perception into kinesthetic images, and translation of kinesthetic images into the final motor patterns that are necessary to produce the construction. Patients do not have to recognize or name the figure; they only have to develop an accurate concept or gestalt. The relationship of angles and sides, orientation on the page, and three-dimensionality must all be appreciated if accurate motor integration is to be carried out. The final step, of course, requires adequate limb strength and coordination.

Constructional impairment, rather than constructional apraxia, will be used to describe the failure to perform adequately on any of these tasks. As implied in the preceding paragraph, a disturbance in praxis (apraxia) is merely a breakdown in the execution of the learned movements that are involved in the constructional task.[9] The term apraxia excludes the component of visual perception and thus does not accurately describe the neuropsychologic complexity of the process. It is true that pure limb apraxia (see Chapter 9) can cause failure, but so can faulty visual perception, spatial orientation, or right-left sense. For this reason, the more inclusive term constructional impairment will be used.

## EVALUATION

As we have mentioned, constructional ability may be tested in a variety of ways. Different levels of performance can often be found in the same patient on different tests. As an example of the range of test materials that may be employed, Warrington[22] has listed the following six basic types of tests that can be used to elicit evidence of constructional impairment: (1) two-dimensional block designs, (2) paper-and-pencil reproduction of geometric shapes, (3) spontaneous drawings, (4) stick-pattern reproduction, (5) three-dimensional block constructions, and (6) spatial analysis tasks that require the patient to shade in the portion of a design that is common to two or more overlapping figures. Patients with brain lesions show differences in the incidence, severity, and quality of constructional impairment, depending upon the type of test used and the nature and location of their lesions.[1,3,19]

The clinical examination of constructional impairment in the individual patient should ideally include several tests to tap somewhat different aspects of constructional ability. Drawings to command and reproduction drawings remain the most easily administered and interpreted tests.

The use of the tests outlined in this book presumes that the patient has adequate vision (20/100, as objectively tested) and sufficient motor ability to effectively use paper, pencil, and blocks. Deficits in either motor or sensory channels can hinder performance. Impairment secondary to these problems does not reflect a disruption in the higher cortical function these tests are designed to assess. A number of constructional tests that include a memory component are available.[4,10,18] Although the inclusion of the memory component does increase the sensitivity of constructional tests, it also raises serious problems in the interpretation of the test results. Deficits in drawings from memory may be due to either memory or constructional problems or to a combination of the two. We feel that memory is a sufficiently important variable that it should be specifically tested in isolation. As we have stressed throughout this examination, a primary goal of each aspect of mental status testing is to assess as discrete a cognitive function as possible. The reader is referred to Appendix 1 for further information regarding the availability and description of visual memory tests.

The following brief tests of constructional ability are included for bedside and office testing. These tests were chosen because of their ease of administration and interpretation, a limited need for apparatus and specialized equipment, and their proven efficacy in the detection of diffuse and focal brain lesions.

## Reproduction Drawings

*Directions.* We suggest that reproduction drawings be administered first when assessing constructional ability, because of their apparent simplicity and familiarity. The drawings presented below are organized in order of increasing difficulty and should be administered in this order. Both two- and three-dimensional drawings are used because of frequent quantitative and qualitative performance differences noted on these two somewhat different tasks. The examiner may either use a standard predrawn set of designs (probably best because the stimuli are identical for each administration and generally of better quality than quickly drawn bedside examples) or draw the stimulus figures on the left side of a piece of blank white paper for each administration. The use of separate sheets of paper for each design is advised for patients who are highly distractible or perseverative. The use of lined progress note forms, consult sheets, and other handy, but perceptually confusing, paper is not recommended. It is often useful to use two colors of pencil or felt tip pen to reduce the possibility of confusion between the drawings of the patient and those drawn by a hurried examiner. Patients who become frustrated with their efforts should be encouraged by the examiner to continue.

Introduce each item by saying "Please draw this design exactly as it looks to you" (Fig. 7-1).

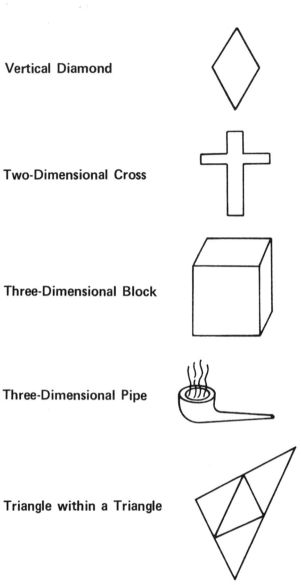

Vertical Diamond

Two-Dimensional Cross

Three-Dimensional Block

Three-Dimensional Pipe

Triangle within a Triangle

FIGURE 7-1. Test items for Reproduction Drawings Test.

*Scoring.* To aid the examiner in quantifying the adequacy of patients' performance on this test, an objective scoring system[15] is provided for rating the relative quality of each drawing.

0—Poor    Given for nonrecognizable reproductions or a gross distortion of the basic design gestalt.

| 1—Fair | Given for moderately distorted or rotated two-dimensional drawings or a loss of all three-dimensionality with moderate distortions or rotations on three-dimensional designs. |
| 2—Good | Given for minimal distortions or rotations with adequate integration on two-dimensional designs and some evidence of three-dimensionality, but less than perfect reproduction on three-dimensional designs. |
| 3—Excellent | Given for perfect (or near perfect) reproductions of two- and three-dimensional drawings. |

Patients' drawings that show evidence of rotations of more than 90 degrees (Fig. 7-2, example 1), perseveration (Fig. 7-2, example 2), or "closing in" (Fig. 7-2, example 3) are given ratings of 0.

Standardization of these designs with nonselected brain-damaged and low-IQ (< 80) normal people has indicated highly significant (p < .0001) differences in performance by the two groups on each design. A rating of 0 on any design resulted in a 100 percent probability of the patient being correctly classified as brain damaged, with a 0 percent probability of misclassification (false-positive). A rating of 1 resulted in an 80 percent probability of brain damage.[21]

Although the physician will soon gain familiarity with this test and develop his or her own scoring criteria based upon experience, examples from our clinical population of poor, fair, good, and excellent drawing reproductions are shown in Figures 7-3 to 7-7 to aid the examiner in rating each design.

## Drawings to Command

*Directions.* The three drawings in Figure 7-8 were selected from those commonly used by neurologists. The patient is required to draw each of the pictures to verbal command. Introduce the test by saying "I would now like you to draw some simple pictures on this paper. Draw each picture as well as you are able. Please draw a picture of a clock with the numbers and hands on it; a daisy in a flowerpot; a house in perspective so that you can see two sides and the roof."

*Scoring.* A simple scoring system similar to that used with reproduction drawings may be used to aid the examiner in quantifying performance on this test.

| 0—Poor | Given for nonrecognizable drawings or a gross distortion of the basic gestalt. |

**Example 1  ROTATION**

**Example 2  PERSEVERATION**

**Example 3  "Closing In"**

FIGURE 7-2. Examples of patient drawings with specific types of errors.

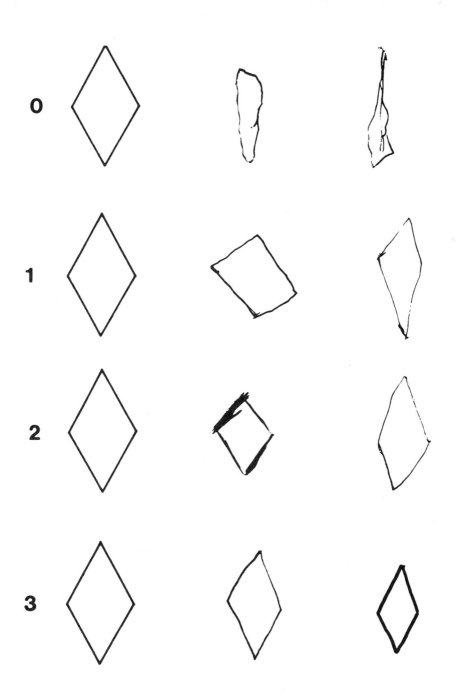

FIGURE 7-3. Renderings of Vertical Diamond Test, with scores of 0 (poor) through 3 (excellent).

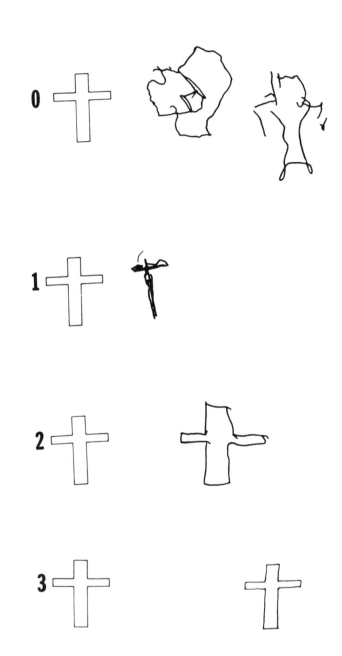

FIGURE 7-4. Renderings of Two-Dimensional Cross Test, with scores of 0 (poor) through 3 (excellent).

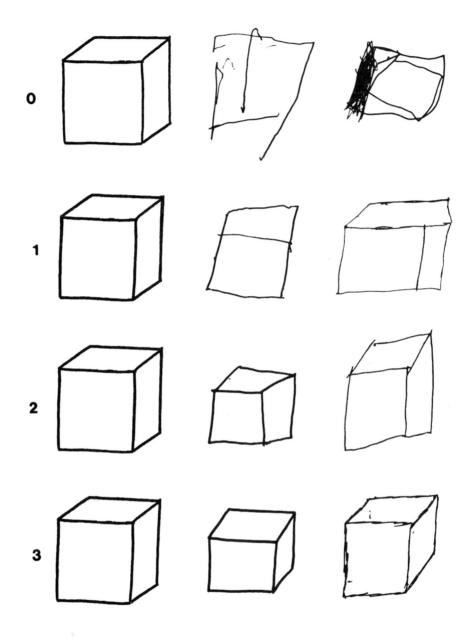

FIGURE 7-5. Renderings of Three-Dimensional Cube Test, with scores of 0 (poor) through 3 (excellent).

FIGURE 7-6. Renderings of Three-Dimensional Pipe Test, with scores of 0 (poor) through 3 (excellent).

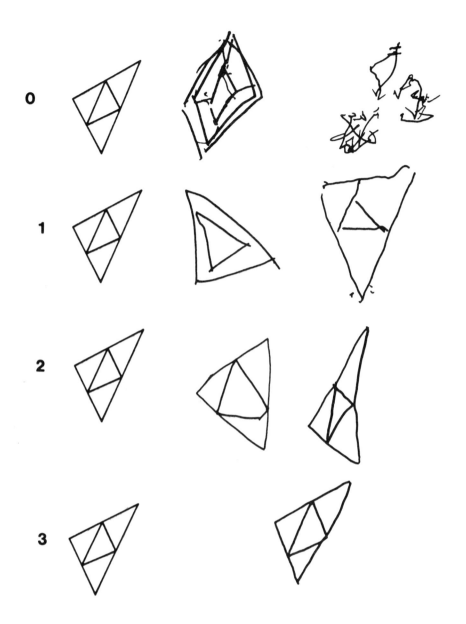

FIGURE 7-7. Renderings of Triangle within a Triangle Test, with scores of 0 (poor) through 3 (excellent).

FIGURE 7-8. Test items for Drawings to Command Test.

| 1—Fair | Given for moderate distortion or rotation of any of the drawings or a loss of three-dimensionality on the house drawing. The clock should contain one of the following: an approximately circular face or the numbers 1 through 12. The daisy should be recognizable as a flower in a pot, and the house should be recognizable as a house. |
|---|---|
| 2—Good | Given for only mild distortions with adequate integration on all pictures. The house should contain some evidence of three-dimensionality. The clock should contain two of the following: circular face, the numbers 1 through 12, or symmetrical number placement. The daisy should be in the generally appropriate shape—a circular center with petals around it. The house should contain the basic elements of a house. |
| 3—Excellent | Given for perfect (or near perfect) representations of the items with all appropriate components, placement, and perspective. The house and flowerpot should be clearly three-dimensional. |

Representative clinical examples of poor, fair, good, and excellent drawings are shown in Figures 7-9 to 7-11 to aid the examiner in rating each picture.

## Block Designs

The following test, although important and often providing excellent clinical data, does require equipment other than paper and pencil and is considered ancillary.

*Directions.* The use of this test requires only four multicolored cubes (obtained from the suppliers of the WAIS-R or from many toy stores as Kohs blocks) and four stimulus designs, which may be drawn with colored pens or pencils on pieces of heavy white paper. The stimulus designs should be accurately drawn in the approximate size of the design completed with blocks. The designs in Figure 7-12 are arranged in ascending order of difficulty. Take four blocks and say "These blocks are all alike. On some sides they are all red; on some, all white; and on some they are half red and half white. I would like you to take these blocks and make a design (or picture) that looks like this picture." If the patient fails to accurately reproduce Design 1, score the response as a failure and demonstrate the correct reproduction. Continue with each design in turn, being sure to mix up the blocks after each effort.

**0**

**1**

**2**

**3**

FIGURE 7-9. Renderings of Drawings to Command Test (clock), with scores of 0 (poor) through 3 (excellent).

114

FIGURE 7-10. Renderings of Drawings to Command Test (flowerpot), with scores of 0 (poor) through 3 (excellent).

**0**

**1**

**2**

**3**

FIGURE 7-11. Renderings of Drawings to Command Test (house in perspective), with scores of 0 (poor) through 3 (excellent).

FIGURE 7-12. Test items for Block Designs Test.

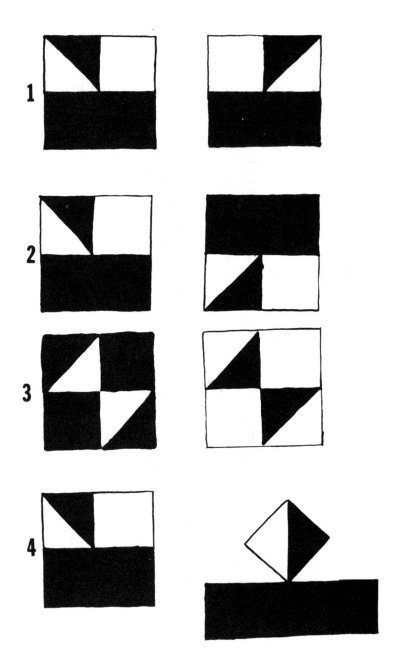

FIGURE 7-13. Examples of common errors on Block Designs Test. (1) Right-left rotation. (2) Near-far rotation. (3) Figure-ground reversal. (4) "Stringing out."

*Scoring.* Only perfect reproductions of the designs are considered correct. Rotations (either right-left or near-far) are scored as incorrect, as are figure-ground (color) reversals. A score of 1 is given for each correctly reproduced design. Perfect reproductions of each design are expected in the normal individual.

Examples of commonly seen rotation, reversal, and "stringing out" errors are shown in Figure 7-13.

A number of specific types of errors on constructional tests are generally accepted as almost pathognomonic of brain damage when made by a nonretarded patient above the age of 10 years. The majority of these errors can be seen on both paper-and-pencil and block-design tests. Of primary importance among these pathognomonic signs are the following:

1. The rotation by more than 45 degrees or the disorientation of the whole figure or a component of it on the background.
2. Perseveration or the repetition of the entire figure or part of it.
3. Fragmentation of the design or the omission of parts of the figure.
4. Significant difficulty in either integration or the placement of individual parts at the correct angles or location.
5. The substitution or addition of "dog ears" for angles on the drawn figure.

The occurrence of any of these errors should raise a strong question of brain dysfunction requiring more detailed evaluation.

## ANATOMY

The parietal lobes are the principal cortical areas involved in visual-motor integration. Visual receptive areas of the occipital lobes and the motor areas of the frontal lobes are necessary for the completion of all of the tests, but it is the association cortex of the parietal lobes that is responsible for the complex integration. The actual localization of the various aspects of construction within the parietal lobes is not established, but it is postulated that visual stimuli are spread from primary sensory area 17 to contiguous secondary association area of the inferior parietal lobule (areas 39 and 40), where associations are made between visual, auditory, and kinesthetic images.[16] Most constructional tasks primarily require the kinesthetic analysis of the visual pattern. The kinesthetic images are then translated into motor patterns in the perirolandic cortex. Drawings to command also require an input from the auditory system. The premotor frontal association cortex would theoretically seem to be very important in these highly skilled fine motor tasks. In fact, only a small percentage of patients with lesions restricted to the frontal lobes have constructional impairment.[7] The parietal lobes seem to be the major areas involved in learning skilled movements; the frontal motor areas appear to be more involved in the pure executive nature of the task. (A more extensive discussion of learned skilled movements is contained in the section on apraxia in Chapter 9.)

## CLINICAL IMPLICATIONS

If a nonretarded adult demonstrates constructional impairment on the tests outlined in this chapter, parietal lobe dysfunction can be strongly suspected. Although lesions in any quadrant of the brain can disrupt constructional performance, the incidence and severity of defects in patients with lesions that are restricted to the frontal lobes are small. Most constructional impairment is seen in patients with cortical damage posterior to the rolandic fissure.[7,13]

At one time, it was felt that the right (nondominant) parietal lobe was actually dominant for constructional ability. Many studies have been performed comparing the relative incidence and severity of constructional impairment in patients with lesions of the right and left hemispheres. These studies clearly demonstrated that performance can be defective with lesions in either parietal lobe.[17] In general, right-hemisphere lesions produce a higher incidence and greater severity of defect than do left-hemisphere lesions.[3] What is certain is that constructional ability is not a function exclusive to the right parietal lobe.[11]

Some subtle differences in qualitative performance that are both interesting and possibly useful in clinical testing have been noted in patients with right and left parietal lobe lesions. On the block designs test, patients with right-hemisphere lesions frequently lose the basic outline of the design and "string out" the blocks.[12] This is shown in example 4, Figure 7-13. These patients tend to make scattered and fragmented drawings that show loss of spatial relations and orientation on the page. Patients with left-hemisphere lesions show more coherent block designs, with maintenance of external configuration but loss of accurate internal detail (example 3, Fig. 7-13). Their drawings tend to be simplifications of the model, lacking detail, but with preserved general spatial relationships. Obvious differences in the performance of the two groups are not always seen, and elaborate scoring schemes have been designed to bring out the subtle differences.[5] Such systems are interesting but are probably not of practical significance to the bedside clinician. Thus, constructional impairment usually suggests right-hemisphere pathology without strong indication of locus within the hemisphere.[14] Without very careful assessment of qualitative performance, it is not always possible, using constructional tests alone, to determine the side of the lesion in the individual patient unless unilateral neglect is present. When a patient's constructional ability is grossly impaired, in the face of normal language, right-hemisphere dysfunction is strongly suggested.

Patients with lesions that are confined to the parietal lobes will often show evidence of significant constructional impairment on mental status testing, yet fail to demonstrate abnormalities on the standard neurologic examination. Therefore, the presence of errors on constructional testing should lead to a more complete neurodiagnostic work-up.

The most dramatic examples of constructional impairment occur in patients with bilateral cortical disease. This is particularly well demonstrated in cerebral atrophy. Patients with Alzheimer's disease (by far the most common dementia) regularly show constructional difficulty as one of the earliest signs of their disease.[20] The patients with multiple infarct dementia, seen in cerebral vascular disease, may also show constructional impairment, but usually they have other abnormal neurologic signs as well. Patients in confusional states from toxic or metabolic factors frequently have constructional impairment during the acute stage. This is secondary to reversible physiologic disturbance of the cortex rather than to structural damage.

Because of the high incidence of constructional impairment in dementia, such tasks are very good screening tests in patients of advancing age who present with vague psychiatric or neurologic complaints.

Standard drawing and other constructional tests are not only useful in the detection of brain disease, but they also have been commonly used by psychologists to evaluate both the maturational stage of perceptual-motor development (constructional ability) and the presence of specific constructional problems in children. The ability to integrate visual stimuli and to construct or draw a reproduction is closely related to both chronologic and intellectual maturation in young children.[2,8,15] Errors in construction, including poor integration of the parts, distortions or simplification, perseveration, and rotations, are common early in development (5 to 7 years) and tend to decrease with age.[6] Relatively errorless performance on simple drawing tests is expected by ages 10 to 12.[15] Measured intelligence tends to be relatively highly correlated with constructional performance in children; for adults of normal intelligence (e.g., IQ above 85), IQ appears to have a limited effect upon constructional ability.[18] Both children and adults with a significant mental deficiency tend to show inferior performance on most constructional tests.[4] Formal studies have indicated that it is difficult, but not impossible, to use drawing tests to differentiate intellectually impaired (e.g., IQ below

70) but socially and vocationally independent adults from similar individuals with demonstrable brain damage.[21]

As with any skilled motor coordination activity, both initial exposure and repeated practice have an effect upon the ability to reproduce paper-and-pencil designs or to complete block constructions. Social deprivation and a lack of academic experience do, therefore, have a detrimental effect upon constructional performance.

The physician who uses constructional tests as a part of the mental status examination must be cautious in interpreting the results of performance by patients with a history of retardation and/or a poor academic background. Placed in the proper interpretative context, however, we feel that drawings and other constructional tests may be fruitfully used with such patients.

## SUMMARY

Constructional ability is a highly developed cortical integrative function that is primarily carried out in the parietal lobes. Drawings and block constructions are easily administered tests to evaluate this function. Impairment of constructional performance usually suggests disease of the posterior portions of the cerebral hemispheres, although other areas of the cortex may be involved. Since constructional ability is so frequently disturbed in brain disease, testing this function is a very important and highly useful component of the mental status examination.

## REFERENCES

1. Arrigoni, G. and De Renzi, E.: Constructional apraxia and hemispheric locus of lesions. Cortex 1:170, 1964.
2. Bender, L.: A Visual Motor Gestalt Test and its Clinical Use. American Orthopsychiatric Association, New York, 1938.
3. Benson, D. F. and Barton, M.: Disturbances in constructional ability. Cortex 6:19, 1970.
4. Benton, A.: Revised Visual Retention Test. The Psychological Corporation, New York, 1974.
5. Benton, A. L.: Visuoperceptive, visuospatial and visuoconstructive disorders. In Heilman, K. M. and Valenstein, E. (eds.): Clinical Neuropsychology. Oxford University Press, New York, 1979, pp. 186–232.
6. Black, F. W.: Reversal and rotation errors by normal and retarded readers. Percept Mot Skills 36:895, 1973.
7. Black, F. W. and Strub, R. L.: Constructional apraxia in patients with discrete missile wounds of the brain. Cortex 12:212, 1976.

8. Frostig, M., Lefever, D., and Whittlesey, J.: A developmental test of visual perception for evaluating normal and neurologically handicapped children. Percept Mot Skills 12:383, 1961.
9. Geschwind, N.: The apraxias: Neural mechanisms of disorders of learned movement. Am Sci 63:188, 1975.
10. Graham, F. and Kendall, B.: Memory for Designs Test. Psychology Test Specialists, Missoula, Mont., 1960.
11. Hécaen, H.: Apraxias. In Filskov, S. B. and Boll, T. J. (eds.): Handbook of Clinical Neuropsychology. John Wiley & Sons, New York, 1981, pp. 267–286.
12. Kaplan, E.: Personal communication, 1973.
13. Kertesz, A.: Right hemisphere lesions in constructional apraxia and visuospatial deficit. In Kertesz, A. (ed.): Localization in Neuropsychology. Academy Press, New York, 1983, pp. 455–470.
14. Kertesz, A. and Dobrowski, S.: Right hemisphere deficits, lesion size and location. J Clin Neuropsychol 3:283, 1981.
15. Koppitz, E.: The Bender Gestalt Test for Young Children. Grune & Stratton, New York, 1964.
16. Luria, A.: The Working Brain. Basic Books, New York, 1973.
17. Mack, J. L. and Levine, R. N.: The basis of visual constructional disability in patients with unilateral cerebral lesions. Cortex 17:515, 1981.
18. Pascal, G. and Suttell, B.: The Bender Gestalt Test. Grune & Stratton, New York, 1951.
19. Piercy, M., Hécaen, H., and Ajuriaguerra, J.: Constructional apraxia associated with unilateral lesions: Left and right cases compared. Brain 83:232, 1960.
20. Sjörgen, T., Sjörgen, T., and Lindgren, A. G. H.: Mörbus Alzheimer and Mörbus Pick: A genetic clinical, and pathoanatomical study. Acta Psychiatr Scand (Suppl) 82:1, 1952.
21. Strub, R. L., Black, F. W., and Leventhal, B.: The clinical utility of reproduction drawings with low IQ patients. J Clin Psychiatry 40:386, 1979.
22. Warrington, E.: Constructional apraxia. In Vinken, P. and Bruyn, G. (eds.): Handbook of Clinical Neurology, Vol. 4, Disorders of Speech, Perception and Symbolic Behavior. American Elsevier, Amsterdam, 1969, pp. 67–83.

# CHAPTER 8

# Higher Cognitive Functions

Attention, language, and memory are the basic processes that serve as building blocks for the development of higher intellectual abilities. These basic functions are necessary, but not sufficient in and of themselves, to execute more complex cognitive functions. By use of the term higher cognitive functions, we refer to the highest level of human intellectual functioning readily assessable by formal testing methods. Included within this category of functions are the manipulation of well-learned material, abstract thinking, arithmetic computations, and so forth. These are complex neuropsychologic functions that are predicated upon the integrity and interaction of more basic processes.

Because they represent the most advanced stages of intellectual development, the higher cognitive functions are often highly susceptible to neurologic disease. The evaluation of these functions in the mental status examination may often demonstrate the early effects of cortical damage before the more basic processes of attention, language, and memory are impaired. The individual's ability to perform effectively within the environment is determined in large part by his or her adequacy in performing these higher-order functions. Accordingly, an assessment of the patient's performance in these areas will provide useful diagnostic information, as well as information concerning social and vocational prognosis.

## EVALUATION

There are many different ways to evaluate the higher cognitive functions; most intelligence tests are largely based upon assessments of these functions. In general, the higher cognitive functions may be categorized in the following hierarchical groupings: (1) the fund of acquired information or the store of knowledge; (2) the manipulation of old knowledge (e.g., calculations or problem solving); (3) social awareness and judgment; and (4) abstract thinking (e.g., the interpretation of proverbs or the completion of conceptual series). The store of basic acquired information is most efficiently assessed by simple verbal tests of vocabulary, general information, and comprehension. Specific examples of these kinds of tests may be seen on any basic intelligence test (e.g., WAIS-R Vocabulary, Information, Picture Completion). General intelligence, education, and social exposure are closely related to performance on these tasks, and the results of any evaluation must be interpreted in the light of this background information. The manipulation of old knowledge is a more active process that involves both an intact fund of general information and the ability to apply this information to new or unfamiliar situations. Questions concerning social comprehension and calculation ability may be used to assess this function. Social awareness may be evaluated by questions concerning the knowledge of environmental situations (e.g., What should a person do if he sees smoke or fire in a grocery store?).

Social judgment is a more complex function that includes the basic knowledge of social situations, the socially appropriate response in such situations, and the ability to personally apply the correct response when faced with a real situation. Because of the real nature of social judgment, it is difficult to assess validly in an abstract test situation. The patient who matter-of-factly states that he or she would calmly inform the manager of smoke or fire in the store when asked the question in the confines of an office or hospital bed may act very differently when faced with the actual situation. Therefore, data concerning the patient's social judgment is best obtained by history from family or other informants who have witnessed the patient's actual performance in dealing with day-to-day events. An alternative possibility, albeit a somewhat cumbersome and inefficient procedure, is to place the patient in actual, but experimental, situations that require an immediate appropriate social response. This method of evaluation is likely to be impractical except in research settings; thus the social history is recommended for practical purposes.

Abstract thinking, which is perhaps the highest level of cognition, may be readily assessed by the use of proverbs, conceptual series, or analogy interpretation.

The following tests are recommended to evaluate a spectrum of relevant higher cognitive functions.

## Fund of Information

*Directions.* The following questions provide a reasonable estimate of the patient's store of knowledge or fund of general information. They are presented in order of increasing difficulty and should be administered in this order. If it is obvious from history or interview that the patient is of above average intelligence, some of the less difficult questions may be omitted. Continue to ask questions until completion of the test or until the patient has failed three successive questions. If the patient's response is unclear, ask him or her to explain more fully. The examiner may repeat the question if necessary, but should not paraphrase the question or spell or explain words that are unfamiliar to the patient.

*Test Items*

| Questions | Acceptable Responses |
|---|---|
| 1. How many weeks are in a year? | 52 |
| 2. Why do people have lungs? | To transfer oxygen from air to blood; to breathe |
| 3. Name four people who have been president of the U.S. since 1940. | Any appropriate presidents |
| 4. Where is Denmark? | Scandinavia |
| 5. How far is it from New York to Los Angeles? | Any answer between 2300 and 3000 miles |
| 6. Why are light colored clothes cooler in the summer than dark colored clothes? | Light colored clothes reflect heat from the sun, while dark colored clothes absorb heat |
| 7. What is the capital of Spain? | Madrid |
| 8. What causes rust? | Oxidation: a chemical reaction of metal, oxygen, and moisture |
| 9. Who wrote the Odyssey? | Homer |
| 10. What is the Acropolis? | Site of the Parthenon in Athens |

*Scoring.* The acceptable response for each question is provided above. The patient's answer must either be exact or very closely approximate the acceptable response. In our experience, the average patient with an adequate educational background should answer a minimum of six questions appropriately. Less adequate performance is indicative of an impaired fund of general information and is suspicious of retardation, limited social and educational exposure, or significant dementia. Conversely, more adequate performance suggests above average intelligence and education.

# Calculations

*Directions.* Calculations are complex neuropsychologic functions that involve the somewhat distinct components of: (a) rote tables (e.g., addition, subtraction, and multiplication); (b) the basic arithmetic concepts of carrying and borrowing; (c) recognition of the signs $(+, -, \times, \div)$; and (d) correct spatial alignment for written calculations. Because these components of calculations may be disturbed in isolation, they are assessed separately in this section. When evaluating calculations, it is important to require the patient to actually calculate and not to merely recite rote tables (e.g., $4 + 4 = 8$ or $3 \times 5 = 15$). This allows the observation of many different types of errors and provides additional clinical data that are important for a description of the nature of the deficit and for providing neuroanatomic implications. Performance on calculation is, of course, closely related to educational experience. Tell the patient, "We are now going to do some arithmetic examples. Some will be familiar to you and some will not. Try your best on each one."

Verbal Rote Examples

Read each example in a clear voice in the following form: "What is 4 and 6?" Record the patient's response.

1. Addition
   $4 + 6 = (10)$
   $7 + 9 = (16)$

2. Subtraction
   $8 - 5 = (3)$
   $17 - 9 = (8)$

3. Multiplication
   $2 \times 8 = (16)$
   $9 \times 7 = (63)$

4. Division
   $9 \div 3 = (3)$
   $56 \div 8 = (7)$

Verbal Complex Examples

Read each example in the following form only once: "What is 8 and 13?" Allow only 20 seconds for a response; a failure to respond within the time, even if a correct response is ultimately given, is scored as a failure. Record the patient's response.

1. Addition
   $14 + 17 = (31)$

2. Subtraction
   $43 - 38 = (5)$

3. Multiplication
   $21 \times 5 = (105)$

4. Division
   $128 \div 8 = (16)$

## Written Complex Examples

Provide the patient with the following written examples and ask him or her to complete the examples. To preclude problems of distractibility and perseveration, it is useful to provide each example on individual cards or to write each new example after the patient completes the previous example. Examples written on a single sheet of paper should be widely separated. Allow a reasonable amount of time for completion of each example. A failure to complete the example within 30 seconds should be noted. Record the patient's response, including problems in alignment.

1. Addition
$$108$$
$$+\ 79$$

2. Subtraction
$$605$$
$$-\ 86$$

3. Multiplication
$$108$$
$$\times\ 36$$

4. Division
$$43\,/\,559$$

*Scoring.* Each response should be scored as correct or incorrect. By comparing performance on each computation subtest, it is possible to determine the patient's overall level of calculation ability and area of adequacy and deficit (e.g., intact rote tables, but unable to complete complex, verbally presented examples). Errors specific to a particular aspect of computation (e.g., division) or to a modality of presentation (e.g., intact performance on verbally presented items and impaired performance on written examples) should be noted. Errors involving borrowing and alignment on written examples should be recorded (Fig. 8-1). If an objective measure of arithmetic is needed, the examiner should refer to a standard achievement test such as the Wide Range Achievement Test.[7]

## Proverb Interpretation

*Directions.* The ability to interpret proverbs accurately requires an intact fund of general information, the ability to apply this knowledge to unfamiliar situations, and the ability to think in the abstract. The following proverbs are presented in ascending order of difficulty. Tell the patient, "I am going to read you a saying that you may or may not have heard before. Explain in your own words what the saying means." Read each proverb exactly as written. Do not paraphrase or otherwise explain

**1**

**2**

**3**
$$\begin{array}{r} 605 \\ -86 \\ \hline \end{array}$$

**4**
$$\begin{array}{r} 63 \\ \times 27 \\ \hline \end{array}$$

FIGURE 8-1. Examples of calculation errors. (1) Patient with a large right-hemisphere lesion and left neglect. (2) Patient with head trauma and a right parietal hematoma. Note poor alignment as well as other calculation errors. (3) Patient with 2 years of college education now shows signs of early dementia. (4) Patient with Alzheimer's disease. Note that rote multiplication is good but there are gross problems with basic arithmetic processes.

130

the proverb. Continue only until the patient fails on two successive proverbs. If the patient's response to the first proverb is concrete, or if he or she is unable to interpret it, the examiner should supply the correct answer and explain that this is the expected type of response.

*Test Items*

1. Don't cry over spilled milk.
2. Rome wasn't built in a day.
3. A drowning man will clutch at a straw.
4. A golden hammer breaks an iron door.
5. The hot coal burns; the cold one blackens.

*Scoring.* The primary scoring criterion for proverb interpretation is the degree of abstraction demonstrated by the patient in explaining the proverb. It is helpful to rate the quality of the patient's response to each proverb. To aid the examiner, examples of abstract (2 points), semiabstract (1 point), and concrete (0 points) responses to each proverb are provided below:

1. Don't cry over spilled milk.
   0—Concrete      "The milk's all over the floor."
                       "When the milk is on the floor, you can't use it."
   1—Semiabstract  "It's gone; don't worry about it."
                       "Don't cry when something goes wrong."
   2—Abstract     "Once something is over, don't worry about it."
                       "Don't be concerned about events that are beyond control."

2. Rome wasn't built in a day.
   0—Concrete      "It took a long time to build Rome."
                       "You can't build cities overnight."
   1—Semiabstract  "Don't do things too fast."
                       "You have to be patient and careful."
   2—Abstract     "If something is worth doing, it is worth doing it carefully."
                       "It takes time to do things well."

3. A drowning man will clutch at a straw.
   0—Concrete      "Don't let go when you're in the water."
                       "He's trying to save himself."
   1—Semiabstract  "Self-preservation is important."
                       "It's a last resort."
   2—Abstract     "A person in trouble will try anything to get out of it."

"If sufficiently desperate, a person will try anything."

4. A golden hammer breaks an iron door.

| | |
|---|---|
| 0—Concrete | "Gold can't break iron!" |
| | "Gold is too soft to break a door." |
| 1—Semiabstract | "Gold's worth more than iron." |
| | "The harder something is, the more you have to work to get it." |
| 2—Abstract | "Virtue conquers all." |
| | "If you have sufficient knowledge, you can accomplish even the most difficult." |

5. The hot coal burns; the cold one blackens.

| | |
|---|---|
| 0—Concrete | "Hot coals will burn you and leave it black." |
| | "Hot coals get black when they're cold." |
| 1—Semiabstract | "You can get trouble from both." |
| | "Getting burned and dirty are both bad." |
| 2—Abstract | "Extremes of anything can be detrimental." |
| | "There may be bad aspects to things that appear good." |

Concrete responses are pathologic in all but the retarded or illiterate patient. The average patient should provide abstract interpretations to at least the first three proverbs and minimally semiabstract responses to the remaining proverbs. Often, uneducated patients will initially give a concrete response, but they can give abstract interpretations when specifically asked if there is another way of explaining the proverb. Such cued responses should be scored as a semiabstract response. A total score of less than five on proverb interpretation is suspicious. A concrete response or an absence of any abstract responses should suggest an impairment of abstract ability.

## Similarities

*Directions.* Verbal similarities require the patient to explain the basic similarity between two overtly different objects or situations. Similarities is a test of verbal abstract ability that requires the analysis of relationships, the formation of verbal concepts, and logical thinking. The following test items are presented in ascending order of difficulty. Tell the patient, "I am going to tell you some pairs of objects. Please tell me how they are similar, or alike. Each pair is alike in some way." Present the first item pair. If the patient provides the appropriate abstract response, say "Good," and proceed with the next item. If the patient mentions a difference between the items, fails to respond, or states that they are different, score the item 0, provide the appropriate response, and continue with item 2. Give no help on succeeding items.

*Test Items*

1. Turnip—Cauliflower
2. Car—Airplane
3. Desk—Bookcase
4. Poem—Novel
5. Horse—Apple

*Scoring.* The response for each item pair may be scored for adequacy. Two points should be given for any abstract similarity or general classification that is highly pertinent for both items in the pair. One point should be given for responses that indicate specific properties of both items in the pair and that constitute a relevant similarity. A score of 0 is given when the response reflects properties of only one member of the pair, differences, generalizations that are not pertinent to the item pair, and failures to respond. Examples of 2, 1, and 0 point responses are provided below:

1. Turnip—Cauliflower
   - 2 points: Vegetables
   - 1 point: Food; they grow in the ground; to eat
   - 0 points: Buy in the store; have calories; wash them

2. Car—Airplane
   - 2 points: Modes of transportation
   - 1 point: Drive them both
   - 0 points: One's in the air and one's on the road

3. Desk—Bookcase
   - 2 points: Articles of furniture
   - 1 point: Household objects; in the living room; put books on them
   - 0 points: Made out of wood; sit at a desk and put books in the bookcase

4. Poem—Novel
   - 2 points: Artistic works; works of art; creative expression; literary works
   - 1 point: Write them both; tell stories; express feelings
   - 0 points: Famous things; study them in school; people like them

5. Horse—Apple

    2 points:    Living things; God's living objects

    1 point:    Both grow; both are food; both need food; part of nature

    0 points:    Horses eat apples; one is big and one is small; we use them

The nonretarded patient with a normal educational background should obtain a score of at least 5 on this test. Any one concrete (0 point) response or a score of less than 5 is strongly suggestive of reduced general intelligence or impaired abstract ability. Concrete responses on easy pairs are pathologic. In general, performance on this test should be compatible with performance on the Fund of Information Test and on the Proverb Interpretation Test. If Similarities and Fund of Information performance are equally impaired, this is suggestive of retardation or educational deprivation rather than a specific deficit in abstract thinking.

## Conceptual Series Completion

*Directions.* The Conceptual Series Completion is another test of verbal abstraction, the ability to solve unfamiliar and complex verbal problems, and the ability to reason at a high level. Tell the patient, "I am going to show you some numbers, letters, or words in series. Each series will be incomplete and needs an additional word, letter, or number to complete it. Each dash (—) calls for either a number or letter to be filled in. Take each item in order, but if you don't understand it, don't spend too much time on any one item." The following sequences are presented to the patient in written form, either on a standard form prepared beforehand by the examiner or written on a sheet of paper by the examiner.

*Test Items*

| Series | Correct Response |
|---|---|
| 1. A B C D __ | E |
| 2. 1 4 7 10 __ __ | 13 |
| 3. AZ BY CX D __ | W |
| 4. tote to snow on spun up stab __ __ | at |
| 5. elephant 87654321 plan 5732 lap __ __ __ | 735 |

*Scoring.* Each response is scored as correct or incorrect using the above scoring criteria. No unique or original interpretations of the correct response are allowed. The average patient should be capable of completing at least three of the five examples correctly. Less adequate performance is indicative of impaired ability to think in the abstract or to reason verbally.

## ANATOMY

The higher cognitive functions are primarily cortical. They are not, however, functions that have been well localized in the way that language or constructional ability has. Abstract thinking, the ability to manipulate old knowledge, calculation ability, and similar functions are probably widely represented in the cortex. Because of this diffuse representation, an impairment of these functions can result from lesions that are located in various parts of the cortex. Impairment is particularly prominent in widespread bilateral disease (e.g., dementia).

It is likely that these higher cognitive functions are more posteriorly than frontally localized. Although a "loss of abstraction" has been traditionally considered an early sign of frontal lobe dysfunction and was described in patients following frontal lobectomies,[8] underlying defects of attention, memory, and perseveration may well account for the observed deficits in higher cognition.[6,9] In a comprehensive review of the literature concerned with the interaction of frontal lesions and cognitive functioning, Teuber[10] concluded that such lesions generally affect intelligence less than lesions located in the more posterior areas of the brain. Black[1] also documented the differential effects of frontal and nonfrontal unilateral lesions upon cognitive functions. This study again verified that these higher cognitive functions are more commonly impaired with posterior lesions.

Verbal reasoning and abstraction are primarily dominant hemisphere functions with very close relationships with language. Thus, dominant hemisphere lesions frequently interfere with these high-level verbal manipulations.

Impaired performance on calculations may be seen with brain lesions that are bilateral or unilateral on either the right or left side.[4] Lesions in somewhat different areas of the brain may cause different types of impaired calculation ability (dyscalculia).[3] Left-hemisphere lesions in the right-handed patient typically result in more severe impairment of calculations than do corresponding lesions of the nondominant hemisphere.[2] A significant dyscalculia often accompanies aphasia. Similarly, dyscalculia is a significant component of the Gerstmann syndrome (described in Chapter 9), which is secondary to a dominant parietal lobe lesion. Specific calculation defects ascribed to focal frontal, temporal, parietal, and occipital lesions have been described.[5] Impaired calculation ability due to focal lesions in the parietal lobes appears to be more common. This type of disorder is characterized by a loss of the ability to understand the meaning of numbers and numerical concepts (e.g., larger or smaller) and by the inability to align numbers correctly on the page due to visual-spatial deficits. The malalignment in complex computations can often be the most striking feature in the dyscalculia seen with parietal lobe lesions.

## CLINICAL IMPLICATIONS

Deficits in higher cognitive functions are most frequently seen in patients with widespread brain disease of any etiology. These deficits may often be the first sign of deterioration in progressive brain diseases such as Alzheimer's disease or subacute sclerosing panencephalitis. Focal dominant parietal lobe lesions may produce defects in verbally mediated functions and must be considered in the differential diagnosis in any patient presenting with a loss of abstract ability or impaired calculations. As discussed previously, lesions of the frontal lobe typically do not interfere with the fund of knowledge, abstract thinking, and problem solving unless other, more basic, deficits are also present (e.g., perseveration or aphasia). Conversely, social awareness and judgment in social situations is often impaired with large frontal lesions.

Significant functional disease, particularly schizophrenia, may result in impaired abstracting ability. Although the concreteness of the schizophrenic patient is frequently different in nature from that of the organic patient (e.g., symbolic interpretations incorporating the patient's delusions), at times the deficit may be indistinguishable from that seen in organic patients.

Because of the close relationship between higher cognitive functions and general intelligence, mental retardation from whatever cause will result in impaired performance on these tests. Educational deprivation will similarly result in substandard performance that is not of diagnostic significance. Accordingly, performance on the tests of higher cognitive function must be interpreted within the context of both educational background and premorbid intelligence. The test of fund of information provides a reasonable estimate of current intellectual functioning, which may be combined with data from the history to furnish this background information.

## SUMMARY

Higher cognitive functions are measures of the patient's reasoning and problem-solving abilities. These functions are often impaired early in brain disease and thereby offer an effective measure for detecting brain disease in patients with relatively intact performance in other areas (e.g., language or constructional ability). Any deficits will be reflected in the patient's inability to function effectively within the environment. Thus, an evaluation of these functions will aid in making a valid social and vocational prognosis.

# REFERENCES

1. Black, W.: Cognitive deficits in patients with unilateral war-related frontal lobe lesions. J Clin Psychol 32:366, 1976.
2. Boller, F. and Grafman, J.: Acalculia: Historical development and current significance. Brain and Cognition 2:205, 1983.
3. Ferro, J. M. and Botello, M. A. S.: Alexia for arithmetical signs: A cause of disturbed calculations. Cortex 16:175, 1980.
4. Critchley, M.: The Parietal Lobes. Edward Arnold & Co., London, 1953.
5. Grewel, F.: Acalculias. In Vinken, P. and Bruyn, G. (eds.): Handbook of Clinical Neurology, Vol. 4, Disorders of Speech, Perception, and Symbolic Behavior. American Elsevier, New York, 1969, pp. 181-194.
6. Hécaen, H. and Albert, M.: Disorders of mental functioning related to frontal lobe pathology. In Benson, D. F. and Blumer, D. (eds.): Psychiatric Aspects of Neurologic Disease. Grune & Stratton, New York, 1975, pp. 137-149.
7. Jastak, J. and Jastak, S.: The Wide Range Achievement Test. Jastak Associates, Wilmington, Delaware, 1978.
8. Rylander, G.: Mental Changes After Excision of Cerebral Tissue: Ejnar Munksgaards Forlag, Copenhagen, 1943.
9. Stuss, D. T. and Benson, D. F.: Neuropsychological studies of the frontal lobes. Psychological Monographs 95:1, 1984.
10. Teuber, H. L.: The riddle of frontal lobe function in man. In Warren, J. and Akert, K. (eds.): The Frontal Granular Cortex and Behavior. McGraw-Hill, New York, 1964, pp. 410-444.

# CHAPTER 9

# Related Cortical Functions

There are several specific disorders of cortical function that have been of great interest to neurologists and neuropsychologists. Most of these functions are related to high-level motor and sensory processing. Apraxia is an example of a high-level motor disturbance; visual agnosia is a high-level perceptual disturbance. These disorders are of some utility in cerebral localization and are of considerable research interest to neurobehaviorists. Because each disorder is relatively discrete, a complete discussion of each disorder, including terminology, evaluation, and clinical implications, will be presented.

## APRAXIA

Apraxia is an acquired disorder of learned movements that cannot be accounted for by elementary disturbances of strength, coordination, sensation, or lack of comprehension or attention.[23] Many textbooks refer to apraxia as a defect in motor planning. Both definitions indicate that apraxia is not a low-level motor disturbance, but a defect in the integrative steps that precede skilled or learned movements. Different types of apraxia have been described based upon the complexity and nature of the task performed.

There is a motor disturbance that is characterized by clumsiness or involuntary grasp reflexes in the limb contralateral to a cortical lesion.[14] This disturbance has been called a limb-kinetic apraxia. Because these patients have difficulty with basic motor control and display abnormal reflexes, their movements do not meet the classic definition of apraxia.

### Ideomotor Apraxia

Ideomotor apraxia is the most common type of apraxia. Patients with this form of apraxia fail to accurately perform previously learned motor acts. Impairment can be seen in buccofacial, upper or lower limb, or trunkal musculature. The inability to carry out such commands as "Show me how you blow out a match" or "Drink through a straw" is called buccofacial apraxia. Difficulty with arm or leg commands such as flipping a coin, saluting, or kicking a ball is called limb apraxia. Difficulty with trunkal commands such as "Bow," "Swing a baseball bat," or "Stand like a boxer" is called an apraxia of whole body movements.

*Evaluation.* There is a hierarchy of difficulty in performing these ideo-motor tasks. The most difficult level requires that the patient perform the action to verbal command (e.g., "Show me how to flip a coin"). This movement must be mimed without the coin and without any nonverbal cues from the examiner. If the patient fails at this level, the examiner performs the action and asks the patient to imitate him or her. Imitation is easier for most patients with apraxia. If the patient again fails, he or she is provided with the real object and again asked to follow the command. Use of the actual object is the easiest task for the apraxic patient, and many, but not all, of the patients who failed on verbal command and imitation will succeed with the concrete task using the real object. The presence of the object gives the patient additional visual and propriocep-tive cues that facilitate performance. There are innumerable possible commands when evaluating praxis. The following are examples that will frequently elicit apraxic movements:

*Buccofacial Commands*

| Commands | Errors |
|---|---|
| "Show me how to": | |
| 1. "Blow out a match" | Difficulty giving short, controlled exhalation; saying "blow"; inhaling; difficulty maintaining appropriate mouth posture |
| 2. "Protrude your tongue" | Unable to stick out tongue; tongue moves in mouth but tends to push against front teeth and not protrude |
| 3. "Drink through a straw" | Unable to sustain a pucker; blowing instead of drawing through the straw; random mouthing movements |

In testing buccofacial praxis, patients can often cue themselves consid-erably by pretending to have the object (match or straw) in their hands. This self-cuing facilitates performance and should be discouraged by gently restraining the patients' hands.

## Limb Commands

| Commands | Errors |
|---|---|
| "Show me how to": | |
| 1. "Salute" | Hand over head; hand waving; improper position of hand |
| 2. "Use a toothbrush" | Failure to show proper grip; failure to open mouth; grossly missing the mouth; using finger to pick teeth; not allowing adequate distance for shaft of toothbrush |
| 3. "Flip a coin" | Movements miming tossing the coin into the air with an open hand; suppinating or pronating the hand as though turning a doorknob; flexing the arm without flipping thumb against finger |
| 4. "Hammer a nail" | Moving hand back and forth horizontally; pounding with fist |
| 5. "Comb your hair" | Using fingers as teeth of comb; smoothing the hair; inexact hand movements |
| 6. "Snap your fingers" | Extension of fingers with patting movements; tapping finger on thumb; sliding finger off thumb with insufficient force |
| 7. "Kick a ball" | Stamping foot; pushing foot along floor; lateral foot movements |
| 8. "Crush out a cigarette" | Stamping foot; kicking foot on floor |

There are occasions in which apraxia will be found unilaterally. Accordingly, commands should be alternated between left and right limbs. Do not have the patients do the same command sequentially with both hands, because visual self-cuing will improve performance on the second trial.

## Whole Body Commands

| Commands | Errors |
|---|---|
| "Show me how to": | |
| 1. "Stand like a boxer" | Awkward arm position; hands at side |
| 2. "Swing a baseball bat" | Difficulty in placing both hands together; chopping movements |

| 3. "Bow" | Any inappropriate trunkal move-ment |
|---|---|

*Clinical Implications.* The ability to perform skilled movements on verbal command is closely associated with the language functions of the dominant hemisphere. Since adequate verbal comprehension is a prerequisite to praxis testing, the area A (Fig. 9-1) must be intact. Once the command is understood, the information spreads to the contiguous supramarginal gyrus (area B, Fig. 9-1), where the words (e.g., "flip a coin") are associated with the kinesthetic memories present in the postrolandic parietal cortex. These sensory memories of the movement are then transferred along pathway C to the premotor area (D), where memory for motor patterns is evoked. The premotor area then directs the pyramidal neurons in the motor strip (E) to actually perform the action. A lesion at any point along this pathway can cause an ideomotor apraxia. Many patients with lesions in this section of the dominant hemisphere will also be aphasic. Accordingly, praxis testing must be very carefully done to ensure that a comprehension deficit is not responsible for the impaired motor performance.

The above paragraph outlines the pathways for praxis in the right hand (controlled by the left motor area). It has been recognized that the apraxic patient also has an apraxia with the left hand. Figure 9-2 illustrates that a command to the right motor cortex for innervation of the left hand is transferred from the left premotor area $(D_1)$ to the right premotor area $(D_2)$ via the anterior callosal fibers $(F_1)$. Any interruption of this pathway will render the left hand apraxic.[22,23,41] This is often called a sympathetic dyspraxia[21] and can be readily demonstrated in the intact left hand of patients with Broca's aphasia with right hemiplegia. Lesions of the anterior corpus callosum $(F_1)$ will cause an isolated apraxia of the left hand; motor and praxis functions of the right hand are intact.[25] The posterior callosal pathway $(F_2-C_2)$, which could theoretically transmit the praxis information to the right premotor area $(D_2)$, obviously does not. Lesions of the right hemisphere rarely result in a significant apraxia of either hand.[13,16]

This anatomic model has been verified clinically and pathologically and firmly establishes that the hemisphere that is dominant for language is also dominant for learning skilled movements.[23] This dominance is obvious because most individuals have a strong hand preference for writing, throwing, and so forth. Since a lesion of the dominant hemisphere causes an apraxia in both hands, it is apparent that the dominant hemisphere exerts a continual guiding role on movements that originate from the nondominant hemisphere.

FIGURE 9-1. The pathways for praxis in the right hand (controlled by the left motor area).

Not all apraxic patients demonstrate a similar degree and type of impaired performance. Some will fail completely on command (even when comprehension of the command is adequate), yet perform perfectly on imitation. Such patients have a type of disconnection syndrome in which verbal input is literally disconnected from motor areas. Visual input, however, is relayed quickly to the motor areas, and the patient can imitate without difficulty. Most apraxic patients who fail on command, however, also have difficulty with imitation. There are some patients with ideomotor apraxia whose disorder is sufficiently severe that they will fail on verbal command, imitation, and in the use of real objects.

Whole body commands can be performed correctly in the presence of obvious limb apraxia. They can often be accurately carried out by patients with severe auditory comprehension deficits as well. The reason for the relative sparing of performance involving whole body commands in some patients is unclear, but it may be due to the fact that these axial movements are under the control of the more widespread extrapyramidal system.[23] As a rule, however, patients with ideomotor limb apraxia will also demonstrate apraxic axial movements.[35]

FIGURE 9-2. The pathways for praxis with anterior corpus callosum lesion.

## Ideational Apraxia

Ideational apraxia is a disturbance of complex motor planning of a higher order than is seen in ideomotor apraxia. It refers to a breakdown in performance of a task that involves a series of separate steps, such as folding a letter, placing it in an envelope, sealing it, and then placing a stamp on it. The patients are often able to perform each individual step of the task in isolation (e.g., folding the paper), but are unable to integrate the parts accurately to complete the sequence. The patients seem to have lost the overall concept of how to go about completing the task. Some investigators define an ideational apraxia as any difficulty in manipulating real objects.[17] We feel that difficulty with object use in simple limb commands (e.g., inability to flip an actual coin) represents a severe ideomotor limb apraxia and not an ideational apraxia.

*Evaluation.* Several simple tasks are used to demonstrate an ideational apraxia:

| Tasks | Errors |
|---|---|
| 1. Folding a letter, placing it in an envelope, sealing it, and placing a stamp on the envelope | Turning paper around without being able to fold it; folding improperly; licking the wrong side of stamp or envelope; inability to place paper in envelope |
| 2. Placing candle in holder, taking match out of box, lighting candle, and blowing out match | Placing candle in holder wick down; inability to place candle in holder; inability to open or close matchbox; striking match on candle; striking wrong end of match; striking candle on matchbox; blowing out candle and not match |
| 3. Opening toothpaste, taking toothbrush from holder, and placing toothpaste on toothbrush | Removing cap from toothpaste and placing cap on toothbrush; putting toothpaste in toothbrush holder; placing toothbrush back in holder with toothpaste on it |

In each of these tasks, the patient can usually perform each part of the series adequately (e.g., striking the match or brushing teeth), but cannot coordinate the individual movements that are necessary to complete the sequence.

*Clinical Implications.* Ideational apraxia is a complex disability that is usually seen in patients with bilateral brain disease. Any diffuse cortical disease, especially those diseases that affect the parietal lobes, may result in an ideational apraxia. Although the patient fails on a specific task (e.g., lighting a candle), it is obvious from watching the patient's performance that his or her failure is the result of a number of cognitive deficits. Many patients have elements of ideomotor apraxia, and almost all have some degree of constructional impairment and spatial disorientation. Memory is frequently faulty and auditory comprehension diminished. One interesting element in the performance of patients with ideational apraxia is their apparent inability to recognize the use of objects. This failure to recognize objects and their use has been called an object agnosia and may be illustrated by the patient who attempts to light a candle by striking it on the matchbox. The ability to do serial ordering is also impaired, and the complex multistep task becomes a confusing group of discrete parts with no logical sequential relationship. The ambiguity and incongruity of the formal test situation also is confusing. The patient does not quite understand exactly what he or she is supposed to do when the doctor brings out a toothbrush and toothpaste and pushes it benignly toward the patient.

Neuropsychologically, ideational apraxia is the culmination of many significant cognitive deficits. Clinically, it results in the patient's inability to effectively manipulate the environment. The patient cannot cook a meal, make a bed, light a cigarette, put a record on the phonograph, or do any of the dozens of everyday activities that we all take for granted. Ideational apraxia is not a finding seen in isolation but is associated with widespread intellectual deterioration.

## RIGHT-LEFT DISORIENTATION

Right-left orientation is traditionally defined as the ability to distinguish right from left on self and in the environment (e.g., on the examiner's body). This ability is basically a capacity for spatial orientation.[8] The application of the verbal labels "right" and "left" to the respective sides of the body is frequently used to test right-left orientation,[26] but this is a linguistic task that does not necessarily test spatial sense. Right-left disorientation may be developmental in nature or may result from either focal or diffuse brain lesions. Although this disorder is interesting and may combine with other deficits to produce Gerstmann's syndrome (discussed later in this chapter), it is of limited clinical utility when seen in isolation.

*Evaluation.* The following outline, which is in ascending order of difficulty, may be used to test for right-left disorientation.

*Test Items*

1. Identification on self
   a. Show me your right foot.
   b. Show me your left hand.
2. Crossed commands on self
   a. With your right hand touch your left shoulder.
   b. With your left hand touch your right ear.
3. Identification on examiner (with examiner facing patient)
   a. Point to my left knee.
   b. Point to my right elbow.
4. Crossed commands on examiner (with examiner facing patient)
   a. With your right hand point to my left eye.
   b. With your left hand point to my left foot.

Most normal persons will successfully accomplish all items without difficulty, although a percentage of the normal population (9 percent of males and over 17 percent of females) has demonstrable difficulty on right-left testing.[42]

*Clinical Implications.* If right-left disorientation is present, it is important to determine if the patient was ever capable of adequately performing such tasks. As previously mentioned, right-left disorientation may be developmental in nature and may also be associated with reduced general intellectual ability.

Aphasic patients may fail on right-left commands because of their primary language disorder. Anomia can cause confusion in the use of the labels "right" and "left." Deficits in auditory retention will interfere with performance on complex commands.

Thus far, clinical and neuropathologic case studies have failed to demonstrate an association between right-left disorientation and any circumscribed brain lesion.[19] If an acquired disorder of right-left orientation is present, the lesion will generally be located in the parieto-temporal-occipital region of the dominant hemisphere.[28] In our clinical experience, right-left disorientation is infrequent with lesions that are restricted to the nondominant hemisphere. This is also substantiated by Critchley's review.[8]

# FINGER AGNOSIA

Finger agnosia is the inability to recognize, name, and point to individual fingers on oneself and on others.[20] This disorder may be most readily demonstrated in reference to the index, middle, and ring fingers.[7] Finger agnosia is similar to right-left orientation in that it may be developmental in nature or may result from either diffuse or focal brain disease. Its clinical utility for localization of cerebral lesions is relatively limited.

## Evaluation

Evaluation of this function can be very extensive; however, this is probably not justifiable for practical purposes. A brief screening should suffice. Patients must have adequate auditory comprehension and must know or be capable of learning the names of the fingers (thumb, index or pointing finger, middle finger, ring finger, and little finger).

*Test Items*

1. Nonverbal Finger Recognition
   *Directions.* With the patient's eyes closed, touch one of his or her

fingers. Have the patient open his or her eyes and ask him or her to point to the same finger on the examiner's hand.
2. Identify Named Fingers on Examiner's Hand
*Directions.* The examiner's hand should be placed in various positions (i.e., palm down on the table facing the patient; hand held vertically in the air with the palm facing the patient; and hand held horizontally in the air with the palm facing the examiner). The examiner should say "Point to my middle finger," and so forth.
3. Verbally Identify (Name) Fingers on Self and Examiner
*Directions.* The patient's and examiner's hands should be placed in the various positions as described above. The examiner points to the patient's index finger and says, "What is the name of this finger?" and so forth.

## Clinical Implications

Patients with finger agnosia usually have lesions of the dominant hemisphere.[30] Left-handed patients or those with strong family histories of left-handedness may exhibit finger agnosia with lesions of either hemisphere. Parieto-occipital lesions tend to be predominant among those causing finger agnosia.[34] As with right-left testing, aphasia will adversely affect verbally mediated performance.

With diffuse disease, finger agnosia may be seen with aphasia, apraxia, right-left disorientation, or general dementia. For those who desire a more comprehensive review of this topic, see Critchley[8] or Kinsbourne and Warrington.[30]

## GERSTMANN'S SYNDROME

Gerstmann's syndrome is a classic, albeit controversial, neurologic syndrome. It consists of four major components: finger agnosia, right-left disorientation, dysgraphia, and dyscalculia. Most patients with this disorder, however, demonstrate additional neuropsychologic deficits, principally constructional impairment or mild aphasia. The syndrome has localizing value; the demonstration of all four elements indicates damage to either the dominant parietal lobe or to bilateral parietal lobes.[36,39,40] The reader who desires further information regarding this syndrome is referred to Benton,[5] Critchley[11] and Strub and Geschwind.[40]

# VISUAL AGNOSIA

Visual agnosia is a rare, acquired neurologic syndrome in which the patient is unable to recognize objects or pictures of objects presented visually. Visual acuity is adequate, mentation is clear, and aphasia is absent.

Two major categories of visual agnosia have been described in the literature. In the first type, actual visual perception of the object is distorted to the point that recognition is impossible. Such patients are unable to name or tell the use of an object when it is shown to them, but can readily name and demonstrate the use of the object when it is placed in their hands. Kinesthetic cues provide sufficient information for recognition. To evaluate for the presence of visual agnosia, ask the patient to verbally identify common objects presented visually. If the patient fails to recognize the object, allow him or her to manipulate the object. If the patient readily identifies the object after manipulation, the defect is in the visual system. It has been postulated that such patients have damage to their visual association cortex bilaterally (areas 18 and 19). This type of visual agnosia (apperceptive visual agnosia) has been reported in a patient with anoxic encephalopathy secondary to carbon dioxide poisoning.[4]

The second variety of visual agnosia is called associative visual agnosia. Patients with this type of agnosia have adequate visual perception but have the visual cortex disconnected from the language area or visual memory stores. Accordingly, they can recognize the object and demonstrate its use, but they cannot name it. When unable to name an object, such patients are also unable to describe its use.[38] The evaluation for this disorder is similar to that for the first type of visual agnosia, except that adequate visual perception must be demonstrated. This can be done with a simple visual matching task. Lesions that cause this associative agnosia are either bilateral, involving the inferior temporal occipital junction and subjacent white matter,[2] or an infarct that destroys the left occipital lobe and the posterior corpus callosum.[31] This is the same lesion that causes alexia without agraphia (see Chapter 4), and in fact, most patients with associative visual agnosia are alexic. For further reading, refer to Critchley,[9] Bender and Feldman,[3] Lhermitte and Beauvois,[31] Albert, Reches, and Silverberg,[1] and Alexander and Albert.[2]

There are two additional types of visual agnosia that deserve mention but will not be fully discussed. Prosopagnosia is an unusual agnosia in which patients are unable to recognize familiar faces. In such cases, the agnosia is so profound that even members of the patient's immediate family are not recognized. The patient will recognize the person, however, upon hearing his or her voice. The mechanism that results in proso-pagnosia is probably a combination of a disturbance of fine visual discrimination and a failure of memory for the discrete category of human faces. The lesions that are responsible for this disorder are usually in the occipitotemporal areas bilaterally. One of the lesions is usually in the right inferior temporo-occipital region.[32] For further references, see De-Renzi and Spinnler,[18] Benton and Van Allen,[6] Meadows,[32] or Damasio, Damasio, and Van Hoesen.[12]

Color agnosia is an inability to recognize colors secondary to an acquired cortical lesion. Two types of color agnosia have been described. There is a specific color-naming disturbance that results from a disconnection of visual input from the language area. This anomia is associated with the syndrome of alexia with agraphia.[24] In this form, there is no damage to the primary language area and no other evidence of aphasia.

The second and more common disturbance of color recognition is actually a defect in color perception caused by bilateral inferior temporo-occipital lesions. These are the same lesions that cause prosopagnosia, and most patients with this type of color agnosia have concomitant prosopagnosia.[33] For further reading regarding this topic, refer to Critchley[10] and DeRenzi and associates.[15]

## Astereognosis

Stereognosis is the ability to discriminate the size and shape of objects and to identify them by touch alone. This is usually tested during the routine neurologic examination by asking the patient to identify several common objects placed in his or her hand (e.g., coin, key, paper clip, and so forth). The patient is tested with the eyes closed and is given one object at a time. The patient is allowed to manipulate the object freely. Each hand is tested individually.[8,27]

The task demands that the patient be able to integrate spatial features and weight and texture in order to identify the object. If a patient has a defect in primary sensation in the hand, failure to identify the object cannot be attributed to astereognosis.

Astereognosis, or a failure of tactile recognition, is usually indicative of a lesion in the anterior portion of the parietal lobe opposite the astereognostic hand.[37] The lesion involves the post-central gyrus. Cases have been reported in which a unilateral lesion, either right or left, can produce a bilateral defect.[8] A rare form of left-hand unilateral astereognosis has been reported in patients with a lesion in the anterior corpus callosum.[25]

# GEOGRAPHIC DISORIENTATION

Geographic orientation is a complex ability that includes the patient's capacity to find his or her way in familiar environments, to localize places on maps or floor plans, and to find his or her way in new environments. A significant geographic disorientation will interfere with the patient's ability to live a normal life. Such patients are unable to travel alone outside of their home and may even become disoriented within their own houses.

## Evaluation

### 1. History Obtained from Family

In evaluating geographic orientation, it is important to obtain historical information regarding the patient's ability to operate in familiar and unfamiliar environments outside of the formal testing situation. Such information is best obtained from family members rather than from the patient.

  a. Does the patient become lost at work, in the neighborhood, or at home?
  b. Has the patient become lost traveling to a less-frequented location (e.g., the inability to locate a restaurant that he or she had not been to in a year)?
  c. Does the patient have great difficulty orienting to new environments?

### 2. Localizing Places on a Map

Map localization is an abstract task that can quickly detect disturbances in geographic orientation. It is also useful when adequate historical information is unobtainable, and it may bring out subtle defects in unilateral attention.[7]

*Directions.* Have the patient draw a map of the United States. If he or she is unable to produce a recognizable representation, the doctor should draw one or provide a suitable outline. Ask the patient to localize the following cities on the map outline.

1. Boston
2. Seattle
3. Miami
4. Los Angeles
5. New Orleans
6. Chicago

*Scoring.* In reviewing the patient's performance, the following factors should be considered: (1) Are coastal cities located on the coast? (2) Are the cities in the appropriate states? (3) Are all cities in one half of the map (either east or west)? (4) Are attempts made to localize all cities?

### 3. Ability to Orient Self in Hospital Environment

Information concerning the patient's ability to orient himself or herself in the hospital may be obtained from nurses' reports and by observing the patient's capacity to find his or her bed, ward, and bathroom. For example, we saw a patient with communicating hydrocephalus and mild dementia who, upon concluding a fifth office revisit, walked confidently into the closet.

## Clinical Implications

Geographic disorientation has been clinically associated with parietal lobe disease,[8] although few good clinicoanatomic studies have been reported. Of the studies available, there is some suggestion that right-hemisphere lesions most frequently cause geographic difficulty.[29] Other studies, however, have failed to support this finding of lateralization and report an approximately equal incidence of geographic disorientation in patients with right- and left-hemisphere lesions.[7]

A consistent finding of clinical utility is that patients with unilateral lesions tend to localize cities on the map toward the side of their lesion (e.g., patients with left parietal lesions tend to place cities toward the west coast on the map outline). This appears to be a result of neglect of the contralateral visual field.[7] A more generalized geographic disorientation is a frequent finding in patients with diffuse cortical disease and may be an early sign of dementing illness.

Geographic orientation is probably not a unitary cortical function but a combination of more basic cognitive processes including visual memory, right-left orientation, visual perception, and spatial neglect. Performance on formal tests of geographic orientation, such as locating cities on a map outline, is closely associated with both general intelligence and social exposure (education).

One must not minimize the devastating effects that geographic disorientation has upon the patient's ability to function effectively in his or her environment. Such patients are typically unable to work, easily become lost in unfamiliar places, and eventually have difficulty with orientation in even familiar settings such as the neighborhood and home.

# SUMMARY

The cortical functions of apraxia, visual and finger agnosia, astereognosis, geographic disorientation, and right-left disorientation are interesting and may be clinically relevant in localizing brain lesions.

# REFERENCES

1. Albert, M. L., Reches, A., and Silverberg, R.: Associative visual agnosia without alexia. Neurology 25:322, 1975.
2. Alexander, M. F. and Albert, M. L.: The anatomical basis of visual agnosia. In Kertesz, A. (ed.): Localization in Neuropsychology. Academic Press, New York, 1983, pp. 393–415.
3. Bender, M. and Feldman, M.: The so-called "visual agnosias." Brain 95:173, 1972.
4. Benson, D. F. and Greenberg, J.: Visual form agnosia. Arch Neurol 20:82, 1969.
5. Benton, A.: The fiction of the Gerstmann syndrome. J Neurol Neurosurg Psychiatry 24:176, 1961.
6. Benton, A. and Van Allen, M.: Prosopagnosia and facial discrimination. J Neurol Sci 15:167, 1972.
7. Benton, A., Levin, H., and Van Allen, M.: Geographic orientation in patients with unilateral cerebral disease. Neuropsychologia 12:183, 1974.
8. Critchley, M.: The Parietal Lobes. Hafner, New York, 1966.
9. Critchley, M.: The problem of visual agnosia. J Neurol Sci 1:274, 1964.
10. Critchley, M.: Acquired anomalies of colour perception of central origin. Brain 88:711, 1965.
11. Critchley, M.: The enigma of Gerstmann's Syndrome. Brain 89:183, 1966.
12. Damasio, A. R., Damasio, H., and Van Hoesen, G. W.: Prosopagnosia: Anatomic basis and behavioral mechanisms. Neurology 32:331, 1982.
13. DeAjuriagurerra, J., Hécaen, H., and Angelerques, R.: Les apraxies: Varietes cliniques et lateralisation lesionnelle. Rev Neurol 102:566, 1960.
14. Denny-Brown, D.: The nature of apraxia. J Nerv Ment Dis 126:9, 1958.
15. DeRenzi, E., et al: Impairment in associating colour to form, concomitant with aphasia. Brain 95:293, 1972.
16. DeRenzi, E., Motti, F., and Nichelli, P.: Imitating gestures: A quantitative approach to ideomotor apraxia. Arch Neurol 37:6, 1980.
17. DeRenzi, E., Pieczuro, A., and Vignolo, L.: Ideational apraxia: A quantitative study. Neuropsychologia 6:41, 1968.
18. DeRenzi, E. and Spinnler, H.: Facial recognition in brain damaged patients. Neurology 16:145, 1966.
19. Frederiks, J.: Disorders of the body schema. In Vinken, P. and Bruyn, G. (eds.): Handbook of Clinical Neurology, Vol. 4, Disorders of Speech, Perception and Symbolic Behavior. American Elsevier, New York, 1969, pp. 207–240.
20. Gerstmann, J.: Some notes on the Gerstmann-syndrome. Neurology 7:866, 1957.
21. Geschwind, N.: Sympathetic dyspraxia. Trans Am Neurol Assoc 88:219, 1963.
22. Geschwind, N.: Disconnection syndromes in animals and man, Part II. Brain 88:585, 1965.
23. Geschwind, N.: The apraxias: Neural mechanisms of disorders of learned movement. Am Sci 63:188, 1975.

24. Geschwind, N. and Fusillo, M.: Color-naming defects in association with alexia. Arch Neurol 15:137, 1966.
25. Geschwind, N. and Kaplan, E.: A human cerebral deconnection syndrome. Neurology 12:675, 1962.
26. Goodglass, H. and Kaplan, E.: The Assessment of Aphasia and Related Disorders, ed. 2. Lea & Febiger, Philadelphia, 1983.
27. Hécaen, H. and Albert, M. L.: Human Neuropsychology. John Wiley & Sons, 1978, pp. 297–303.
28. Hécaen, H. and DeAjuriaguerra, J.: Meconnaissances et Hallucinations Corporelles. Masson et Cie, Paris, 1952.
29. Hécaen, H. and Angelerques, R.: La Cecite Psychique. Masson et Cie, Paris, 1963.
30. Kinsbourne, M. and Warrington, E.: A study of finger agnosia. Brain 85:47, 1962.
31. Lhermitte, F. and Beauvois, M.: A visual-speech disconnection syndrome. Brain 96:695, 1973.
32. Meadows, J.: The anatomical basis of prosopagnosia. J Neurol Neurosurg Psychiatry 37:489, 1974.
33. Meadows, J.: Disturbed perception of colours associated with localized cerebral lesions. Brain 97:615, 1974.
34. Nielsen, J.: Gerstmann syndrome: Finger agnosia, agraphia, confusion of right and left, and acalculia. Arch Neurol Psychiatry 39:536, 1938.
35. Poeck, K., Lehmkuhl, G., and Willmes, K.: Axial movements in ideomotor apraxia. J Neurol Neurosurg Psychiatry 45:1125, 1982.
36. Roeltgen, D. P., Sevush, S., and Heilman, K. M.: Pure Gerstmann's syndrome from a focal lesion. Arch Neurol 40:46, 1983.
37. Roland, P. E.: Focal increase of cerebral blood flow during stereognostic testing in man. Arch Neurol 33:543, 1976.
38. Rubens, A. and Benson, D. F.: Associative visual agnosia. Arch Neurol 24:305, 1971.
39. Strub, R. L. and Geschwind, N.: Gerstmann syndrome without aphasia. Cortex 10:378, 1974.
40. Strub, R. L. and Geschwind, N.: Localization in Gerstmann syndrome. In Kertesz, A. (ed.): Localization in Neuropsychology. Academic Press, New York, 1983, pp. 295–321.
41. Watson, R. T. and Heilman, K. M.: Callosal apraxia. Brain 106:391, 1983.
42. Wolf, S. M.: Difficulties in right-left discrimination in a normal population. Arch Neurol 29:128, 1973.

# CHAPTER 10

# Summary of Examination

Throughout this book, we have emphasized the importance of performing a systematic and complete mental status examination. Although it is not always necessary to exhaustively evaluate every aspect of mental functioning, there are certain critical functions that should be assessed in every patient. These include level of consciousness, physical appearance and emotional status, attention, expressive and receptive language, memory, constructional ability, and abstract reasoning. Items that are adequate for evaluating these areas are starred in the composite mental status examination (see Appendix 2). With practice, an adequate screening examination can be completed in 15 minutes.

The systematic mental status examination usually allows the clinician to accurately differentiate patients with organic brain disease from normal persons and those with functional disorders. In many cases, it is also possible to specify the type, locus, and degree of disease. For example, knowledge of specific patterns of aphasia often permits the examiner to localize a lesion within the dominant hemisphere. In other cases, the pattern of performance is suggestive of a specific disease entity (e.g., Alzheimer's disease).

In general, the more clinical data the physician obtains regarding the patient's level of functioning in a variety of areas, the better the physician will be able to arrive at the correct diagnosis. Accordingly, the full mental status examination as outlined in this book should be administered whenever feasible. An examination that includes all of the items discussed in this book and outlined in Appendix 2 can be completed in less than an hour. Although all of the data is valuable, the busy physician may not always be able to spend this much time on all routine consultations. In most clinical settings, the physician is initially interested in making a tentative diagnosis and then planning an appropriate diagnostic evaluation. When the physician understands the mental examination, he or she will be able to tailor the examination to fit the clinical situation. Usually, within a few minutes the physician will be able to tell whether significant organic mental changes exist and, if so, what the most likely diagnosis would be.

For example, one of the most common organic brain diseases is dementia.[2] Alzheimer's disease/Alzheimer's senile dementia is the most prevalent and well known of these diseases.[2,3] It is important to recognize the early features of this syndrome because early diagnosis can prevent serious social and vocational embarrassment to both patient and family. The early features of this disease, which can readily be demonstrated on a systematic mental status examination, are apathy, vague subjective complaints, memory difficulties, constructional impairment, and problems with abstract reasoning. As the disease progresses, anomia, apraxia, agnosia, geographic disorientation, and significant deficits in judgment typically appear. There is also a worsening of those defects seen in the early stages of the disease. In the deteriorated stage, all deficits are accentuated, behavior is regressed, language, memory, and thought processes are severely disturbed, and the patients require total care. The diagnosis of Alzheimer's disease in the advanced stages is usually made without difficulty. However, it is surprising how often mild but significant dementia goes unrecognized by family and physician alike.

When necessary, the mental status examination for a patient with suspected dementia can be shortened, but it should include the following essential components:

1. Level of Consciousness: Patients with simple atrophic dementia (Alzheimer's and senile Alzheimer's disease) are fully alert unless they have a secondary decrease in the level of consciousness from medication, medical illness, or focal brain lesion with increased intracranial pressure.
2. Behavior Observations: These are important and will be made throughout the history and examination and will rarely prolong the examination time.
3. Language: Spontaneous speech and comprehension can be roughly assessed during history taking, but repetition and naming should be specifically tested. Although naming and word-finding errors are often present in dementia, repetition is usually intact unless the disease is advanced or there is an associated left-hemisphere lesion with aphasia.
4. Memory: Memory is a critical item. Orientation should be tested first. If the patient fails, particularly if it is a significant failure, this strongly suggests a new-learning/recent-memory deficit. Next,

tell the patient the correct date and location and ask him or her to remember it. Then ask about recent news items for a few minutes, and then ask the orientation questions again. If there is a second failure, in our experience the patient has a significant memory problem and additional testing will only support this initial impression and will not provide additional substantive data. If the patient is oriented or quickly learns his or her orientation, test the patient with the four words test; this is the most valid of the new-learning tasks.

5. Drawings: These take only a few minutes to perform and are an invaluable aid in diagnosing brain disease, especially dementia.
6. Abstract Functions:
   A. Calculations: These are very useful when evaluating demented patients; several examples should be included.
   B. Proverbs and Similarities: These are also useful, and several of each should be asked. The demented patient tends to answer in a very concrete manner.

This screening exam for dementia is very accurate, and after some experience, it should not take more than 15 minutes.

A history of a rapid decrease in mental status (hours to a few days) does not usually suggest a primary dementia, but more likely represents a delirium (acute confusional state). As discussed in Chapter 2, this condition is usually easily recognized by its typical behavioral features and represents a specific diagnostic entity. Further mental status testing will be abnormal, but it rarely adds additional useful diagnostic information.

The preceding two examples of a shortened examination technique are but two of the ways in which valuable diagnostic information can be obtained by tailoring the mental status examination to the individual patient's clinical problem. In patients for whom the history is vague regarding the behavioral complaints or when emotional features predominate, it becomes increasingly important that the examiner perform a more extensive examination.

In the Clinical Implications sections of each chapter in this book, we have attempted to describe many neurobehavioral syndromes as they relate to specific areas of cognitive deficit. Examples of these are the acute confusional states (see Chapter 2), aphasias and related language disorders (see Chapter 5), amnesias (see Chapter 6), and the frontal lobe syndrome (see Chapter 2). These Clinical Implications sections of the book are not intended to be a comprehensive review of neurobehavior or an intensive discussion of any one syndrome. They are, rather, illustrations of the bridge between the data and the diagnosis. See Strub and Black[4] for a complete discussion of these topics. A description of two common patterns of cognitive impairment that illustrate how findings from the mental status examination can lead to a neurologic diagnosis appear below.

## DOMINANT-HEMISPHERE LESIONS

Patients with lesions of the dominant hemisphere will frequently show abnormalities of language functions. In the right-handed patient, evidence of aphasia, alexia, or agraphia almost always indicates left-hemisphere disease. The Gerstmann syndrome, constructional impairment, verbal memory difficulties, ideomotor apraxia, dyscalculia, and impairment of verbal reasoning are all findings that can be seen with left-hemisphere lesions. Denial and neglect are not commonly seen in these patients. Even left-handed patients will frequently show the above findings with left-hemisphere disease, although there is a higher frequency of bilateral representation of the above functions in these patients.

## NONDOMINANT-HEMISPHERE LESIONS

Most patients with lesions of the nondominant hemisphere will not show evidence of language disorders. They do have a more dramatic constructional impairment than patients with dominant-hemisphere lesions. Denial and neglect are more common and severe in degree, malalignment is seen in writing and calculations, and deficits are present in nonverbal memory.

## CONCLUSION

As stated in our introduction, we have intended to help the clinician to understand many of the cognitive functions that can be easily tested at the bedside. We have, hopefully, given enough information concerning these functions and their disturbance in brain disease to allow the examiner to test the patient and to delineate the deficits. Understanding these deficits and how to test for them, and recognizing the common pattern in disease, frequently allow the examiner to make a specific diagnosis.

This mental status examination is qualitative in nature. The neurologist, psychiatrist, psychologist, or general physician, after reading this book, should be able to conduct a comprehensive examination of the patient with brain disease and use the data for diagnosis.

In contrast to this comprehensive qualitative examination, there are some screening tests (the "mini-mental state"[1] being the most widely used) that will give the examiner a single score that is used to identify the presence and degree of organic disease. This quantitative method can provide only a gross estimate of the patient's global cognitive functioning and is very restricted in its contents and scope. This test has a total possible score of 30 points, of which 10 points are given for general orientation, 8 points for rather complex language items, 5 points for serial sevens, 3 points for immediate verbal recall, 3 points for remembering the same verbal items, and only 1 point for copying a rather complex geometric design (interlocking pentagons). Our fear is that the combination of an objective cutoff score with the narrow range of abilities tapped by this test may result in an overconfidence in the test's ability to accurately describe and diagnose patients with known or suspected brain disease. We do not feel that professionals in the field of behavior (i.e., neurologists, psychiatrists, psychologists, and so forth) should rely on this type of gross screening test; rather, they should utilize the more complete and clinically useful examination as outlined in this book.

## TEST DATA RECORDING

As with any medical examination, it is very important to record both what was specifically tested and the patient's responses to each item. To aid in recording these data, a form similar to the composite in Appendix 2 should be used. At the completion of the examination, the clinician should synthesize the data and then summarize and emphasize the key areas of impairment. This summary allows an identification of deficit patterns and the efficient communication of essential findings.

## SUMMARY OF FINDINGS

After completion of the examination, the clinician must summarize and organize the data in such a way that he or she can arrive at the following four clinical implications:

1. Describe the major areas of impairment. Indicate those areas of mental status functioning that are deficient compared to the level

expected in the patient based on his or her education and premorbid function. This implies a deficit in a general area of functioning (e.g., verbal memory, abstraction, or construction ability) rather than an abnormality on an individual test (e.g., paired associate learning). This is the initial step in organizing the data so that it can be interpreted neurobehaviorally.

2. Make a tentative neurobehavioral diagnosis. Having indicated the major areas of impairment, the clinician is now in a position to analyze the pattern of deficits and to make a specific neurobehavioral diagnosis: delirium, dementia, organic amnesic state, aphasia, nondominant hemisphere syndrome, and so forth. The interpretation of the mental status findings is difficult and, as in all fields of medicine, requires clinical experience with patients who have organic brain syndromes (neurobehavioral disorders), as well as additional reading in this area.

3. Arrive at a tentative localization of the lesion. This step is of both practical and academic importance. In a practical sense, findings that suggest a single focal lesion (e.g., fluent aphasia without other deficits—left temporal or temporoparietal) require a far different neurodiagnostic evaluation than does the identification of an acute confusional state. Academically, it is of great interest to attempt to correlate clinical findings with what is known about brain function.

4. Make a tentative clinical diagnosis. This is the final step in the diagnostic process. It requires the clinician to correlate historical and examination data with medical knowledge to make a specific medical diagnosis. As examples: A patient with a slowly developing cognitive deterioration whose mental status examination shows multiple areas of impairment suggesting bilateral brain disease (dementia) yet a normal standard neurologic examination will most likely have Alzheimer's disease. Similarly, an elderly patient with the acute onset of aphasia with fluent paraphasic speech with impaired comprehension (Wernicke's aphasia) probably has had a left middle cerebral artery occlusion.

This entire summary process requires careful thought and considerable clinical knowledge. When the examiner becomes proficient with the examination and familiar with the organic syndromes, this complex process of data analysis and diagnosis becomes easier.

The final steps in any patient evaluation include communicating test findings to the patient, the patient's family, and the referring physician; referring the patient for further evaluation when necessary; and arranging for appropriate subsequent patient management.

# REFERENCES

1. Folstein, M. F., Folstein, S. E., and McHugh, P. R.: "Mini-Mental State": A practical method for grading the cognitive state of patients for the clinician. J Psychiatr Res 12:189, 1975.
2. Katzman, R.: The prevalence and malignancy of Alzheimer's disease. Arch Neurol 33:217, 1976.
3. Katzman, R. and Karasu, T.: Differential diagnosis of dementia. In Fields, W. (ed.): Neurological and Sensory Disorders in the Elderly. Stratton Intercontinental Medical Book Corp., New York, 1975, pp. 103–134.
4. Strub, R. L. and Black, F. W.: Organic Brain Syndromes: An Introduction to the Neurobehavioral Disorders. FA Davis, Philadelphia, 1981.

# CHAPTER 11

# Further Evaluations

After completion of the routine mental status examination, there are a number of situations in which additional evaluation is warranted. This section will briefly discuss the contributions of the neuropsychologist, speech pathologist, and psychiatrist in the total evaluation of the patient with organic brain disease. Despite the important contributions of such specialists, it is beyond the scope of this book to offer more than an introduction and suggested readings.

## NEUROPSYCHOLOGY

The clinical neuropsychologist is trained at the Ph.D. level, with either a 1-year clinical internship or a post-doctoral fellowship in which formal training is given in the use of standard psychologic tests and specialized procedures to evaluate patients with organic brain disease. Their training generally includes neuroanatomy, physiology, and basic clinical neurology, in addition to topics of a more traditional psychologic nature. The clinical neuropsychologist is primarily concerned with the identification, quantification, and description of changes in behavior that are associated with brain dysfunction. By reason of specialized training, the clinical neuropsychologist's area of interest and expertise is the relationships between human behavior (whether specific to a response on a formal test or in general) and brain function. Accordingly, he or she can aid in a variety of important clinical problems, including differential diagnosis, lateralization and localization of lesions, establishment of baselines of behavior and cognitive performance from which improvement or deterioration can be gauged, determination of competence in the aged or demented, and development of remedial methods for the rehabilitation of the individual brain-damaged patient.[14,17,19,22]

The neuropsychologic evaluation is a comprehensive, objective assessment of a wide range of cognitive, adaptive, and emotional behaviors that reflect the adequacy (or inadequacy) of cortical functioning. In essence, the neuropsychologic evaluation is a greatly expanded and objectified mental status examination. The mental status examination is designed to briefly screen a variety of critical areas; the neuropsychologic evaluation assesses a wider range of performance in more depth over a longer period of time (2 to 6 hours). It differs from the mental status examination in that it generally uses tests and evaluation procedures that have been standardized with samples of either normal people or brain-damaged patients. Because of this use of standardized measures, comparisons can be made of the individual patient's performance with that of standard groups, as well as the varying adequacy of the same patient's performance across a variety of test areas. The objective and highly quantified nature of most neuropsychologic tests aids in the detection of subtle changes in performance over time (e.g., the slowly deteriorating dementia or the improvement in specific functions after neurosurgery). Because of the wide range of performance assessed and the depth in which it is evaluated, the neuropsychologic evaluation may detect subtle deficits not apparent on the mental status examination.

The neuropsychologic evaluation has a number of advantages not shared by many standard neurodiagnostic techniques. It is noninvasive and has no risk of mortality or morbidity; these factors make the evaluation appropriate for patients for whom the risk of invasive procedures (angiography or contrast CT scan) is too great or for whom the probability of positive findings is sufficiently small that any risk is too high (e.g., the child with soft neurologic signs of "minimal brain dysfunction" on general clinical examination). The neuropsychologic tests are interesting to most patients and do not produce the potential complications of anxiety and pain of some invasive procedures. The evaluation also provides important descriptive and prognostic information that other techniques cannot. This is especially true with regard to a description of the effects of neurologic disease upon the patient as a person and its probable impact upon academic, social, and vocational adjustment.

The physician without ready access to a trained neuropsychologist may, nonetheless, benefit from evaluations performed by clinical psychologists who have had experience in evaluating patients with brain damage. This is especially true if the referring physician is familiar with the types of data provided by the psychologist and knows how to interpret the reports. A review of the information contained in this section and in the appendix of psychologic tests should greatly aid in this interpretation.

A common feature of the psychologic reports that are provided by persons other than neuropsychologists and that may be difficult to interpret without some knowledge of its meaning is the frequent reporting of so-called "organic signs." Such signs typically include the following:

1. Verbal-performance discrepancies (e.g., appreciable differences between the Verbal IQ and Performance IQ on the Wechsler series of intelligence tests). Differences exceeding 25 points are statistically significant,[6] while differences of 15 points are of some clinical utility in identifying neurologic dysfunction.[4,5] Reported verbal-performance discrepancies must be cautiously interpreted in the light of the overall psychologic test profile, any primary sensory or motor deficit (e.g., a visual impairment or cerebral palsy), and the patient's educational background.

2. A scattering of performance levels on the various subtests of the Wechsler tests or among any scores obtained from the full psychologic test battery (e.g., a subtest score of 12 on the WAIS Vocabulary Subtest and 6 on the Similarities Subtest). Such differential performance does indicate discrepant intellectual functioning that should be explained. The physician should recognize, however, that a number of factors (social, psychologic, and educational) other than brain damage may result in such subtest "scatter." Accordingly, this sign should not be interpreted in isolation as indicating brain damage.

3. An indication of visual-motor dysfunction as detected by any measure of constructional ability, including the nonverbal WAIS subtests, the Bender Gestalt test, drawings to command, and so forth. The best predictors of brain damage on such tests are specific errors of rotation and perseveration. Errors that are related to the integration of parts or the distortion of the gestalt tend to be maturational rather than pathologic. Constructional ability and its impairment are covered in depth in Chapter 7. Suffice it to say, a wide variety of social, maturational, motor, and sensory factors, as well as brain damage, may impinge upon constructional ability; thus, information regarding performance in this area must be evaluated within the context of the total psychologic evaluation and the patient's history.

In sum, the information provided by the clinical psychologist may be valuable to the physician in describing the abilities and disabilities of the patient and in helping to make a diagnosis of brain damage. The referring physician must, however, utilize the services of a well-trained and experienced psychologist, must understand something of the nature of the commonly employed psychologic tests, and must be able to interpret both the utility and the limitations of the so-called brain damage indicators or "organic signs."

## Referral

Appropriate referrals for neuropsychologic evaluation include patients in whom brain damage is suspected but not unequivocally verified, as well as those for whom the physician requires further information regarding diagnosis, description of the effects of a well-verified lesion upon behavior, or prognosis and management. As with any consultation, the referring physician should state as clearly as possible what question(s) he or she needs answered (e.g., "Is this patient demented or depressed?" or "Will this head injury interfere with the patient's ability to do his or her job?").

Cognitive and behavioral disturbances may occur in the absence of any clear-cut physical signs of cerebral disease on a standard clinical neurologic examination; this is particularly true in cases of early dementia. Dementia typically presents with vague behavioral complaints such as mental dullness, concentration problems, increasing apathy and loss of interest in job or family, chronic fatigue, depression, and memory problems. The neuropsychologic evaluation of such patients can often contribute to an early diagnosis. The common diagnostic problem of differentiating between dementia and depression is frequently solved by the data obtained in the neuropsychologic battery. In other cases, the neuropsychologic evaluation may also provide data suggestive of brain dysfunction and may serve as a basis for ordering more extensive and specific neurodiagnostic procedures.

The evaluation can also determine the relative impact of the organic and functional components in a patient with both neurologic and psychiatric complaints.

Any patient with a documented brain lesion should receive a complete neuropsychologic evaluation as part of the rehabilitation program. The comprehensive nature of the evaluation can provide valuable information regarding the effect of the lesion upon cognitive functioning, emotional status, behavior, and social adjustment. Objective data will elucidate both specific areas of impairment and residual abilities. This outline of strengths and weaknesses is valuable for describing the effects of specific neurologic lesions upon the individual patient and provides information that is critical for vocational and social rehabilitation.

Periodic reevaluation can provide reliable objective information regarding the speed and degree of recovery after brain injury or after neurosurgical procedures. Similarly, repeated evaluations can be used to assess deterioration in cases of progressive disease or to rule out such progression in equivocal cases. Preneurosurgical and postneurosurgical testing will help to quantify the effects of surgery upon the cognitive, behavioral, vocational, and social functioning of the patient. In a similar sense, the effects of any medical treatment (e.g., the use of levodopa in parkinsonism or anticonvulsants in epilepsy) can be well documented by pretreatment and posttreatment neuropsychologic evaluation. These changes over time are difficult to assess without an adequate baseline of data encompassing a wide range of behavior.

It is obvious that in any case of trauma or suspected brain damage involving litigation or compensation, the objective data obtained from neuropsychologic evaluation are of great value in documenting and describing the presence, absence, or degree of disability. There is considerable legal precedent for the admission of testimony of psychologists as expert witnesses in such cases.[15]

## Neuropsychologic Evaluation

Below is a summary of the clinical services that can be provided by the neuropsychologist.

*Categorization.* This section provides information regarding the presence or absence of brain dysfunction and the presence or absence of significant emotional disturbance. The differential diagnosis of a primary organic or a primary functional disorder is made. If significant components of both organic and functional features are present, the relative impact of the two will be discussed.

*Localization.* Typically, performance on the neuropsychologic test battery can be analyzed to provide data to determine if the brain dysfunction is diffuse or focal. Further analysis provides data regarding the lateralization of the lesion in the right or left hemisphere and localization of the lesion in the anterior or posterior region of the hemisphere.

*Description.* Information included in this category pertains to a comprehensive description of the patient's current level of functioning in a wide range of cognitive, adaptive, personality, and behavioral areas. The patient's premorbid level of functioning can usually be estimated from the academic and social history and an analysis of the variability of performance on various tests. From comparisons of the estimated premorbid level of functioning and current performance on standard tests, a relatively accurate indication of deterioration in any of the areas assessed by the battery can be made. A comprehensive overview of the patient's deficits and residual abilities is made in order to provide a description of current functioning, to explain present behavior, to determine the relative effects of organic and functional factors, and to provide a baseline of data from which to judge future change. Answers to the question of mental competence and social independence can also be provided by data obtained in the neuropsychologic evaluation.

*Prognosis and Recommendations.* Based upon the nature of the neurologic disease and the pattern and degree of deficits seen during the neuropsychologic evaluation, a determination of the probability and degree of expected recovery can be made for many patients. As previously mentioned, serial evaluations some months apart greatly aid the ability to make valid prognostic statements in case of either deterioration or recovery. Finally, recommendations for further ancillary evaluations, including psychiatric, speech pathology, occupational therapy, and social service, are made when warranted. Recommendations regarding specific remedial methods or programs may also be made.

*Components of the Neuropsychologic Evaluation.* The specific tests employed in a neuropsychologic evaluation battery will vary with the age of the patient and the nature of the problems, the specified referral questions asked by the referring physician, and the particular training and experience of the psychologist. Virtually all such test batteries will, however, include assessment of the following functions:

1. History: developmental, educational, vocational, and social
2. Behavior: attention, mood, rapport, and motivation
3. Intelligence: including general intelligence, verbal intelligence, and nonverbal intelligence
4. Language: including auditory discrimination, single word and sentence comprehension, repetition, and various aspects of expressive language
5. Memory: including verbal and nonverbal memory, immediate recall, recent and remote memory, incidental memory, and new-learning ability
6. Abstract reasoning: including verbal and nonverbal reasoning, learning to learn, and conceptual shifting
7. Spatial analysis and constructional ability: including paper-and-pencil reproduction, three-dimensional constructions, reproduction from memory, and visual analysis not requiring a motor response
8. Perceptual ability: including visual, auditory, and tactile perception
9. Geographic orientation
10. Time orientation
11. Achievement in reading, spelling, and calculations
12. Perceptual motor speed: including planning ability and concept manipulation
13. Motor strength and coordination
14. Personality
15. Social functioning

Using the data that were generated by the neuropsychologic evaluation, the psychologist typically uses five stages of inference to reach conclusions regarding the patient's neuropsychologic functioning. These include:

1. Levels of performance compared with standard norms (e.g., IQ of 67, with 100 as norm)
2. Levels of present performance compared with known or estimated premorbid levels (e.g., memory quotient of 74 in a practicing lawyer)
3. Variability of performance in tests of different cognitive functions (e.g., IQ of 108 (70th percentile) and progressive matrices below the 10th percentile)
4. Discrepancies between tests subsumed by the two hemispheres (e.g., Finger Tapping Test performance of 25 with the right dominant hand and 44 with the left hand)
5. Presence of pathognomonic signs (specific behavioral deficits present only with brain dysfunction) (e.g., paraphasic speech or unilateral neglect)

References to specific tests that assess these functions and result in these inferences are listed in Appendix 1.

In sum, we have found that neurologists and neuropsychologists can beneficially work closely together and make mutually rewarding contributions in the evaluation, description, and management of patients with cognitive and behavioral changes secondary to organic brain disease.

The literature pertaining to clinical neuropsychology has increased almost exponentially since the publication of the first edition of this book. The amount of available material forces the interested reader to be highly selective in choosing books that are both current and clinically pertinent. The state of the art in 1974[19] can now be viewed as an early stage in the proliferation of relevant publications. The following should be considered to be a selective sampling from the available literature: Filskov and Boll,[7] Heilman and Valenstein,[9] Horton and Wedding,[10] and Lezak.[14]

## SPEECH PATHOLOGY

Patients with significant difficulty in communicating should be evaluated by a speech pathologist. All such patients will not be treatment candidates; however, by means of a thorough language evaluation, the speech pathologist is best able to determine appropriate candidates for rehabilitation and to provide other services to patients who are not selected for treatment. Patients with aphasia, apraxia of speech, or dysarthria are examples of primary neurologic patients who are appropriate for referral. The speech pathologist should be an important member of any comprehensive rehabilitation team; this is particularly true when a unit sees a large number of stroke patients. Functional speech and language disorders such as elective mutism and hysterical aphonia are ideal conditions for speech evaluation and treatment. Evaluation by the speech pathologist provides a description of the patient's level of communication, the possible benefits of therapeutic intervention, and a plan for family counseling to facilitate alternate methods of communicating with the patient.

Virtually every physician has access to speech pathologists either in private practice or in hospital, university, or community clinics. The speech pathologist may be trained at either the master's or doctoral level. The American Speech and Hearing Association and many states issue licenses or certificates of clinical competence to qualified clinicians. Referring physicians should ensure the basic clinical competence of any speech pathologist they consult. Many speech pathologists will have specialized knowledge and experience in treating patients with articulation disorders, stuttering, or aphasia. The evaluation and treatment of aphasia is a very specialized field, and physicians should determine the speech pathologist's competence in this area before referring aphasic patients.

## Referral

The major reasons for referring patients to a speech pathologist include:

1. The mental status examination indicates a communication disorder that requires a more thorough evaluation.
2. Obvious communication disorders that require a screening evaluation to determine the appropriateness of speech therapy.
3. The significant communication disorder that requires family counseling to inform the family members about the patient's problem and to assist in maximizing communication in the home. This may include alternative modes such as sign language or communication boards/computers.

The physician may see the following general types of speech and language problems that require more comprehensive evaluation than can be provided in the office:

1. Articulation disturbances such as the dysarthrias seen in pseudo-bulbar palsy, bulbar paralysis, neuromuscular disease such as myasthenia gravis, cerebellar disorders, cerebral palsy, and basal ganglia disease such as parkinsonism.
2. Functional (hysterical) aphonias, especially in patients with histories of minor trauma or surgery to the throat or vocal cords.
3. Elective mutism.
4. Dysfluency (stuttering). This disorder is seen in both children and adults and, if untreated, may pose a significant obstacle to successful social and vocational adjustment.
5. Patients with acquired language disorders (aphasia, alexia, agraphia) deserve an initial speech and language evaluation, both to determine the potential for speech therapy and to aid the patient's family in understanding and dealing with the communication disorder.
6. Patients with buccofacial apraxia in the presence or absence of aphasia may benefit from speech evaluation and therapy directed toward articulation and the intelligibility of speech, as well as other buccofacial activities such as drinking and swallowing.

## Speech and Language Evaluation

The comprehensive speech and language evaluation can be expected to provide information regarding the following:

*Diagnosis.* A definition of the primary language disorder (e.g., nonfluent aphasia, dysarthria, buccofacial apraxia, and so forth).

*Description.* A comprehensive description of the type of language disorder, including all areas of deficit (e.g., word-finding problems, alexia, or auditory comprehension problems) and residual language abilities. The description should contain some quantitative index of the degree of the problem in each area assessed to allow comparison with subsequent evaluations. Some statement should be made regarding the effect of the language deficit upon the patient's communication ability in formal (test or interview) and informal (social) areas.

*Recommendations.* Is speech therapy indicated? If so, what will be the emphasis of the therapy? What will be the frequency of therapy visits? What is the projected duration of therapy? What are the specific plans for home therapy by family members and for family counseling?

*Goals of Therapy and Prognosis.* What are the primary goals of speech and language therapy? What is the prognosis for language recovery? What will be the long-term social impact of the language disorder?

*Components of the Speech and Language Evaluation.* There are numerous systems and methods of speech and language evaluation. The system and the specific tests employed will be determined partly by the needs of the particular patient and partly by the individual speech pathologist's training and experience. Because the enumeration of these methods is beyond the scope of this book, the interested reader is referred to the following texts and manuals: Albert and associates,[1] Goodglass and Kaplan,[8] Kertesz,[12] Porch,[18] Sarno,[20] and Spreen and Risser.[23]

A comprehensive evaluation should include the following elements:

1. An examination of the oral physiology, including the strength and coordination of the muscles of articulation
2. A description of the characteristics of speech articulation—dysarthria, dysfluency, and dysprosody
3. A description of apraxias if present, both verbal (speech) and nonverbal (nonspeech facial movements)
4. An evaluation for aphasia, specifically including an assessment of verbal comprehension, repetition, and word-finding ability, and a description of spontaneous speech
5. An assessment of reading and writing
6. An evaluation of the adequacy of nonverbal communication, including an assessment of the patient's ability to communicate utilizing gestures or other methods regardless of the language deficit
7. A description of the patient's general behavior and specific behavioral responses to the stress of language items

## Treatment

Treatment is not universally efficacious in all speech and language disorders.[21] The following is a general breakdown of the expected results with a number of patient types based upon our clinical experience.

Excellent results can often be produced in rehabilitating patients with (1) functional voice disorders, exclusive of elective mutism (which is more resistant to traditional forms of speech therapy); and (2) mild to moderate articulation problems.

Good results can be expected in patients with (1) anomic aphasia, (2) oral apraxia, and (3) moderate articulation problems.

Fair results are generally obtained in patients with (1) Broca's aphasia, (2) moderate to severe articulation problems, (3) aphasia with mild to moderate comprehension defects, and (4) elective mutism (unless intensive behaviorally oriented therapy is employed, in which case the prognosis is improved).

Poor results are typical in therapeutic efforts with patients with (1) global aphasia, (2) Wernicke's aphasia, (3) severe dysarthria and oral apraxia, and (4) language disturbances secondary to dementia.

It is emphasized that these are general statements of prognosis; the individual patient with a particular language disorder will not always respond to therapy as projected. Accordingly, a speech and language evaluation of the patient with any developmental or acquired communication disorder is important to provide the opportunity for therapy to patients who may benefit from it.

## PSYCHIATRY

Many patients with organic brain disease will have an associated emotional disturbance that requires psychiatric consultation. Patients referred for psychiatric evaluation include those with psychiatric disorders that preceded their neurologic problem, those with emotional reactions to brain disease (e.g., reactive depression), patients in whom an emotional reaction complicates dementia, and those with functional disorders that present as neurologic conditions (e.g., hysterical paralysis).[3]

Emotional factors are significant in the rehabilitation and social reintegration of any patient with organic disease. Therefore, a psychiatrist should be consulted to aid in the management of any patient with an emotional disturbance that is severe enough to interfere with rehabilitative efforts or home adjustment.

### Referral

Because of the relatively high incidence of both mental illness and brain disease, many patients will have coexisting psychiatric and neurologic conditions (e.g., a brain tumor in a schizophrenic patient, or a seizure patient with a manic-depressive disorder). As a specific example, we saw a 37-year-old woman with a long psychiatric history. The patient was also an alcoholic and over the years had sustained several significant head injuries. After alcohol withdrawal, she had several grand mal seizures and was admitted to the neurology ward. As her postictal confusion cleared, she demonstrated gross delusional and aggressive behavior. After a complete history and medical evaluation, we determined that the patient had an acute neurologic condition superimposed upon a pre-existing schizophrenia. Because of the significant psychosis, psychiatry was consulted for treatment and long-term management.

It is not uncommon for emotionally stable individuals to develop a significant emotional reaction to a recent neurobehavioral disorder such as aphasia. Depressive reactions, anxiety, paranoia, and aggressiveness may develop in response to brain damage. Such emotional reactions may significantly interfere with rehabilitation efforts. As an example, a 62-year-old woman developed a right hemiplegia and anomic aphasia secondary to a cerebral thrombosis. After the acute stage, she became increasingly depressed to the point of apathy, self-deprecation, and constant crying. She would no longer actively participate in physical therapy and appeared to abandon any hope of improvement. When a serious emotional reaction such as this is superimposed on an organic deficit, the emotional component must be treated in conjunction with the medical treatment.

Demented patients present a particular challenge because they have both intellectual and emotional changes as a part of their disease. These changes produce a variety of difficult management problems that are often best handled with the aid of a psychiatrist. In the early stage of dementia, patients may retain considerable insight; this capacity to realize the seriousness of their condition often results in profound depression. Other dementing patients are unaware of their deteriorating intellectual ability; such patients often push themselves beyond their capability and thus develop frustration and severe anxiety. This situation was aptly illustrated by a recent case: A 58-year-old businessman was referred because of failing memory. His examination revealed a genuine memory deficit and other evidence of an early dementia. Severe anxiety was prominent and interfered with both specific test performance and his social and vocational life. This anxiety was greatly reduced by restructuring his lifestyle (e.g., his wife helped him with his business; he discontinued many civic duties; and he used a mild tranquilizer to sleep). After several months, retesting showed improvement and he was better able to carry out his home and job responsibilities. Anxiety or depression can greatly exacerbate the mental and social disability experienced by the demented patient. The psychiatrist can provide great assistance through the use of psychotropic drugs, family counseling, and general patient management.

The diagnostic problem of differentiating among dementia, depression, and dementia with depression is both common and difficult in clinical practice. Because this differential diagnosis is critical in terms of patient management and treatment, the psychiatrist should be involved early in the evaluation process. The misdiagnosis of depression as dementia will deprive the patient of appropriate treatment and leave the family with the erroneous impression that the disease is progressive and irreversible. Conversely, the misdiagnosis of dementia as depression may lead to ineffective and costly psychotherapy, leave the patient subject to the social and vocational problems resulting from intellectual deterioration, and mislead the family as to the prognosis of the disease.

Psychiatric referral is also indicated for patients who develop depression in response to or as a part of a chronic neurologic disease such as myasthenia gravis, epilepsy, multiple sclerosis, or parkinsonism. These patients frequently live long and productive lives if they are able to accept and deal with their disabilities in a realistic fashion.

Many patients with chronic organic brain syndromes such as aphasia, dementia, traumatic encephalopathy, or Korsakoff's disease become management problems and eventually require long-term care in a psychiatric hospital. Early referral to the psychiatrist or psychiatric social worker can help the family and the physician with the administrative and legal details involved in institutionalization.

A final group of patients who may initially be seen by the neurologist but who require referral to the psychiatrist are the patients with hysterical conversion reactions. Many patients will present with symptoms that mimic neurologic disease (e.g., limb paralysis, loss of speech, or sensory loss) but demonstrate no organic etiology. The treatment for such functional disorders is psychotherapy.

## Evaluation

The psychiatrist utilizes psychiatric interview techniques, a psychiatrically oriented mental status examination, and personality tests in the evaluation. Information on specific interview and evaluation techniques is readily available in all major psychiatric texts.[2,11,13,16,24]

## Treatment

Even though specific treatment is frequently unavailable for the primary brain disease, behavioral and pharmacologic treatment can improve the lives of many of these patients.

Medication is particularly useful in patients with pre-existing psychiatric disease. In such patients, the underlying psychiatric disorder will respond to a standard regimen of psychotropic medication. Antianxiety or mood-elevating drugs are effective in treating the anxiety or depression frequently seen as a reaction to organic brain disease. Major tranquilizers are often required to control the agitation and nocturnal wanderings of the deteriorated organic patient.

Standard psychotherapeutic methods can be used in some organic patients who retain comprehension, memory, and insight. On the other hand, insight therapy would be useless in many patients (e.g., severe amnesics, demented patients, those with significant frontal lobe behavioral changes, and Wernicke's aphasics). In this latter group of patients, behavior modification techniques aimed at specific behaviors are more appropriate and successful.[25]

Family counseling is often the most useful form of patient management. Through discussion, the psychiatrist is able to help the family understand the patient's problem and to offer suggestions on management. With the psychiatrist's help, the family can then restructure the patient's routine in an effort to minimize environmental stress.

The medical-legal aspects of organic disease are also very important and must be part of a long-term management program. The patient's competence to make a will, to conduct personal financial affairs, and to enter into contracts such as marriage should be established in each case.

Finally, every treatment plan should include a consideration of possible eventual full-time supervision if the patient becomes unmanageable in the home. The details of nursing home or institutional placement should be worked out with the help of the psychiatrist, social worker, and the patient's family. Such plans should be considered early in the course to allow time to assess the family's financial and personal resources; to determine the availability of home nursing services, nursing homes, and institutions; and to preclude the necessity of unsatisfactory and hasty decisions made at a time of crisis.

## SUMMARY

The management of patients with organic brain disease is a multidisciplinary effort. Physicians are strongly encouraged to acquaint themselves with the services offered by their colleagues in related specialized fields. With this effort, physicians will be able to better understand their patients and to provide them with more comprehensive care.

## REFERENCES

1. Albert, M. L., et al: Clinical Aspects of Dysphasia. Springer-Verlag, New York, 1981.
2. American Psychiatric Association: Diagnostic and Statistical Manual of Mental Disorders (DSM III). American Psychiatric Association, Washington, D.C., 1980.
3. Benson, D. F. and Blumer, D. (eds.): Psychiatric Aspects of Neurologic Disease, Vol. II. Grune & Stratton, New York, 1982.
4. Black, F. W.: WISC verbal-performance discrepancies as indicators of neurological dysfunction in pediatric patients. J Clin Psychol 30:165, 1974.
5. Black, F. W.: WAIS verbal-performance discrepancies as predictors of lateralization in patients with discrete missile wounds. Percept Mot Skills 51:213, 1980.

6. Field, J.: Two types of tables for use with Wechsler's intelligence scales. J Clin Psychol 16:3, 1960.

7. Filskov, S. B. and Boll, T. J. (eds.): Handbook of Clinical Neuropsychology. Wiley-Interscience, New York, 1981.

8. Goodglass, H. and Kaplan, E.: The Assessment of Aphasia and Related Disorders, ed. 2. Lea & Febiger, Philadelphia, 1983.

9. Heilman, K. M. and Valenstein, E. (eds.): Clinical Neuropsychology, ed. 2. Oxford University Press, New York, 1984.

10. Horton, A. M. and Wedding, D.: Clinical and Behavioral Neuropsychology. Praeger Scientific Press, New York, 1983.

11. Kaplan, H. I. and Sadock, B. J.: Modern Synopsis of Comprehensive Textbook of Psychiatry III. Williams & Wilkins, Baltimore, 1981.

12. Kertesz, A.: Aphasia and Associated Disorders: Taxonomy, Localization, and Recovery. Grune & Stratton, New York, 1979.

13. Kolb, L. C. and Brodie, H. K.: Modern Clinical Psychiatry. WB Saunders, Philadelphia, 1982, pp. 184-225.

14. Lezak, M. D.: Neuropsychological Assessment, ed. 2. Oxford University Press, New York, 1983.

15. McMahon, E. A. and Satz, P.: Clinical neuropsychology: Some forensic applications. In Filskov, S. B. and Boll, T. J. (eds.): Handbook of Clinical Neuropsychology. Wiley-Interscience, New York, 1981, pp. 686-701.

16. Novello, J.: The psychiatric history and mental status examination. In Novello, J. (ed.): A Practical Handbook of Psychiatry. Charles C Thomas, Springfield, Ill., 1974, pp. 40-48.

17. Parsons, O.: Clinical neuropsychology. In Speilberger, C. (ed.): Current Topics in Clinical and Community Psychology, Vol. 2. Academic Press, New York, 1970, pp. 1-60.

18. Porch, B.: Porch Index of Communicative Ability. Consulting Psychologists Press, Palo Alto, Calif., 1967.

19. Reitan, R. and Davison, L. (eds.): Clinical Neuropsychology: Current Status and Applications. John Wiley & Sons, New York, 1974.

20. Sarno, M. T. (ed.): Acquired Aphasia. Academic Press, New York, 1981.

21. Sarno, M. T.: Recovery and rehabilitation in aphasia. In Sarno, M. T. (ed.): Acquired Aphasia. Academic Press, New York, 1981, pp. 485-529.

22. Satz, P. and Fletcher, J. M.: Emergent trends in neuropsychology: An overview. J Consult Clin Psychol 49:851, 1981.

23. Spreen, O. and Risser, A: Assessment of aphasia. In Sarno, M. T. (ed.): Acquired Aphasia. Academic Press, New York, 1981, pp. 67-127.

24. Stevenson, I. and Sheppe, W.: The psychiatric examination. In Arieti, S. (ed.): The American Handbook of Psychiatry, Vol. 1. Basic Books, New York, 1959, pp. 215-234.

25. Wells, C. E. and Duncan, G. W.: Neurology for Psychiatrists. FA Davis, Philadelphia, 1980.

# Standard Neuropsychologic Tests

The purpose of this section is twofold: (1) to briefly introduce the physician to those tests that are commonly encountered in neuropsychologic reports on patients evaluated because of known or suspected brain dysfunction, and (2) to give the interested psychologist an annotation and source listing for those tests and procedures that are either representative of those frequently used in neuropsychology or that have proven their clinical utility to the authors. It is not intended as a comprehensive overview of neuropsychologic procedures or an intensive evaluation of any individual technique. See Lezak[54] for such a presentation.

Letters in parentheses following test names refer to the following publishers and distributors. Other sources can be found in the references to specified tests.

## TEST PUBLISHERS AND DISTRIBUTORS

A. American Guidance Service
   Publishers' Building
   Circle Pines, Minnesota 55014
B. Consulting Psychologists Press
   577 College Avenue
   Palo Alto, California 94306
C. Jantak Associates, Inc.
   1526 Gilpin Avenue
   Wilmington, Delaware 19806
D. Lea and Febiger
   600 South Washington Square
   Philadelphia, Pennsylvania 19106

E. Neuropsychology Laboratory
University of Victoria
Victoria, British Columbia V8W 242 Canada

F. Psychological Assessment Resources, Inc.
P.O. Box 98
Odessa, Florida 33556

G. The Psychological Corporation
757 Third Avenue
New York, New York 10017

H. Psychological Test Specialists
Box 1441
Missoula, Montana 59801

I. Reitan Neuropsychology Laboratory
1338 East Edison Street
Tucson, New Mexico 85719

J. Stoelting Co.
1350 South Kostner Avenue
Chicago, Illinois 60623

K. Western Psychological Services
12031 Wilshire Boulevard
Los Angeles, California 90025

## SCREENING TESTS

Those clinical psychologists who wish to screen for the possibility of
neurologic problems during a routine evaluation may include one of the
following tests in their evaluation: The Neuropsychological Screening
Exam[68] is a psychometrically oriented mental status examination that
evaluates a number of neurobehavioral functions in a "brief" (40 to 60
minutes) period, yielding a "cutting" score to estimate the probability of
dysfunction. In contrast, the Adult Neuropsychological Questionnaire[62]
and the Neuropsychological Status Examination[69] consist of structured
interviews that are used to collect historical and current complaint data
that can be used to suggest the presence of problems requiring more
extensive evaluation. The Neuropsychological Impairment Scale[65] is a
50-item self-report screening test designed to identify neuropsychological symptoms and deficits. Preliminary research[63,64] suggests that it is
reasonably sensitive, valid, and reliable when used for its stated
purpose—brief screening.

None of these tests is capable of doing more than increasing the suspi-
cion of neuropsychologic dysfunction. They do not replace the need for
doing more comprehensive testing; they do not identify "brain dam-

aged" patients; and they cannot provide the data necessary for a description of the patient's present neuropsychologic status. As a screen, they can be used if properly employed by an experienced clinician.

## Comprehensive Neuropsychologic Batteries

### Halstead-Reitan Battery (I)

This battery includes a well-standardized series of tests of cognitive and adaptive ability. It was originally introduced by Halstead,[37] revised and standardized by Reitan and associates,[14,22,75,77,89] and statistically refined by Russell and associates[80] and others.[89] Its primary limitations include its length, the minimal emphasis on important areas such as memory and language, and a lack of descriptive data that is functionally relevant to the non-psychologist. Augmented by the addition of tests of general cognitive ability, language, and memory, this battery is currently one of the best standardized methods of identifying patients with brain damage.[54]

### Luria's Neuropsychological Investigation (K)

Christensen[17] organized some of Luria's materials and techniques into card form, with a manual of administration instructions, in a framework that corresponded to his conceptualization of brain function-behavior relationships. This contribution allowed the use and adaptation of Luria's experimental procedures for patient examination. The battery includes techniques that assess math functions, auditory-motor organization, kinesthetic functions, higher visual functions, receptive and expressive language, reading and writing, arithmetic skill, memory, and intellectual processes. It is limited in the testing of attention and vigilance, visual memory, and nonverbal abstract reasoning. Its advantage is its ready adaptability to meet the needs of each individual case. However, its lack of normative data restricts the interpretation of some items to a very well-trained and highly experienced examiner.

### Luria-Nebraska Neuropsychological Battery (K)

This battery,[29,30] which is an attempt to standardize and provide normative data on selected items taken from the Christensen-Luria materials, has been the source of both considerable clinical popularity and major criticism in the literature since its inception. Golden and his colleagues[29,30] have uniformly reported the battery's excellent ability to differentiate brain-damaged patients from both normal people and psychiatric patients, while others have concluded that the battery is not diagnostically reliable.[1,20] Reviews of the positive and negative findings with the Luria-Nebraska can be found in Spiers[84] and Stambrook.[87] As of this writing, this battery may have some potential as a comprehensive neuropsychologic instrument, but this is a potential that has not yet been realized.

## Neuropsychologic Test and Laboratory Manuals

(Listed in Alphabetical Order)

Benton, A. L., et al: Contributions to Neuropsychological Assessment: A Clinical Manual. Oxford University Press, New York, 1983.[11]

Kimura, D. and McGlone, J.: Neuropsychology Test Procedures. DK Consultants, London, Ontario, 1983.[49]

Matthews, C. G.: Neuropsychology practice in a hospital setting. In Filskov, S. B. and Boll, T. J. (eds.): Handbook of Clinical Neuropsychology. Wiley-Interscience, New York, 1981, pp. 645–685.[60]

Swiercinsky, D.: Manual for the Adult Neuropsychological Evaluation. Charles C Thomas, Springfield, Ill., 1978.[89]

Tites, R. L.: Neuropsychological Test Manual. Royal Ottawa Hospital, Ottawa, Ontario, 1977.[94]

# TESTS OF INTELLIGENCE

## Leiter International Performance Scale (K)

The LIPS is a measure of intelligence that utilizes a pictured stimulus–block matching paradigm for use with nonverbal children and adults.[52,53] Although not well standardized for validity and reliability at the higher levels (ages 14 to adult), it is a useful adjunct in those situations when a purely nonverbal test is needed.

## Stanford-Binet (Houghton Mifflin)

The S-B[91] is an age-graded, highly verbal test with a wide variety of subtests that are arranged in order of difficulty (and, ostensibly, mental age). It can be used with patients from age 2 through adulthood. Designed primarily for use with children, it is not a part of most neuropsychologic batteries. Another disadvantage is the global nature of the test; only an overall IQ can be obtained. Pattern analysis is deficient and has questionable validity. Its main application for the neuropsychologist dealing with adults is with very low functioning patients who do not have language dysfunction.

## Wechsler Adult Intelligence Scale—Revised (WAIS-R) (G)

The WAIS-R[97] represents the latest revision and standardization of the Adult Wechsler Scales. The test, which has become the standard for the clinical assessment of intelligence for patients between 16 and 74 years of age, provides data that reflect global intellectual functioning (full scale IQ), verbal and nonverbal performance (verbal and performance scale IQs), and subtest performance in the following areas:

| *Verbal Scale* | *Performance Scale* |
|---|---|
| Information | Picture Completion |
| Digit Span | Picture Arrangement |
| Vocabulary | Block Design |
| Arithmetic | Object Assembly |
| Comprehension | Digit Symbol |
| Similarities | |

Use of the WAIS-R with neurologic patients allows an analysis of performance at several levels of inference that are valuable in neuropsychologic assessment: comparisons of individual performance with normative and clinical samples, comparisons of current performance with premorbid functioning, and analyses of intraindividual performance on subtests that assess different areas of cognitive functioning (e.g., verbal vs. nonverbal or verbal-comprehension vs. perceptual-analytic vs. attention-concentration).[82] A Spanish language version of the test that was standardized in Puerto Rico is available,[35] as is the Wechsler Intelligence Scale for Children—Revised[96] for use with patients under the age of 16. More comprehensive reviews of the neuropsychologic use of the Wechsler Scales may be found in Golden and Vicente,[31] Matarazzo,[59] Lezak,[54] and Lawson, Inglis, and Stroud.[51]

## TESTS OF MEMORY

### Wechsler Memory Scale (WMS) (G)

The WMS[95] is a relatively brief (approximately 30 minutes) series of tests that assess a rather disparate group of memory-related functions: (1) personal and current information, (2) orientation, (3) mental control (i.e., attention and concentration), (4) logical memory paragraphs, (5) digit span, (6) visual reproduction from memory, and (7) paired associate learning. Performance on the subtests is summed and statistically age-corrected to provide a memory quotient (MQ), which in some ways is analagous to a full scale IQ (mean = 100, SD = 15). For many years, the major advantage of the WMS was its sheer existence as the only widely available and standardized objective test of memory for clinical use. The test's limitations have been recognized for some time and include its highly verbal nature; an overemphasis on very basic processes, such as personal information and mental control; the procedure of combining widely variable tests to provide a so-called "memory" quotient; and the procedure of age correction for increasing chronological age—which frequently results in test scores that are not reflective of the patient's actual deficits.[28,54] Despite its conceptual and psychometric limitations, the Wechsler Memory Scale continues to be widely used, especially by clinical psychologists.

## Russell Revision of the Wechsler Memory Scale

Russell[79] selected the logical memory paragraphs and visual reproduction subtests for the WMS and devised new administration and scoring procedures. Each subtest is first administered and scored according to standard directions, to be followed 30 minutes later by a delayed recall trial. This technique results in: (1) a short-term memory score, (2) a 30-minute delayed recall score (determined by the same scoring system), and (3) a retained memory score obtained by the formula:

$$\frac{\text{Delayed Recall}}{\text{Immediate Recall}} \times 100$$

This adaptation has proven effective in discriminating between normal people and dementia patients[57] and is useful for comparing verbal with visual memory and delayed with immediate recall in both experimental and clinical settings.

## Randt Memory Test (from authors)

Randt and colleagues[15,70,71] have designed a brief (20 minutes) test battery to objectively assess memory acquisition, storage, and retrieval. The test is theoretically and psychometrically superior to other clinical memory batteries and has the added value of a 24-hour delayed recall. It shares the WMS's verbal emphasis, with disproportionately fewer sensitive measures of nonverbal memory. The Randt is still in the phase of full standardization, although early clinical and experimental work suggests that it will become a useful component of the neuropsychologic evaluation.

## Benton Visual Retention Test (BVRT) (G)

The BVRT[9] consists of several series of simple and complex line drawings that are presented to the patient for varying periods (5 to 10 seconds, depending on the administration form). The patient either reproduces the designs directly or after a variable delay (immediate recall or a 15-second delay). This test, which was designed to assess visual perception and analysis, short-term visual memory, and constructional ability, has explicit scoring instructions and robust normative data. It is useful with a wide age range and has repeatedly proven effective in clinical situations.[58]

## Memory for Designs (H)

This test[34] consists of 15 line drawings of variable complexity that are displayed to the patient one at a time for 5 seconds. Immediately after termination of exposure, the patient reproduces the design. An objective scoring system is provided; however, the procedures contain questionable methods (e.g., totally forgotten designs are not considered, and there is an overemphasis on rotated or reversed reproductions), thus reducing the clinical utility of the tests. Studies of the efficacy of the MFD to detect brain-damaged patients do not generally support its usefulness when compared with similar tests.[40]

## Recurring Figures Test (from author)

The Recurring Figures Test designed by Kimura[48] assesses visual recognition memory and rate of forgetting. The patient is initially presented with a set of 20 geometric and irregularly drawn nonsense figures that include eight stimulus designs. The patient is then shown a pack of 140 designs comprised of 7 sets of the original 8 designs interspersed with 84 unique designs. The patient is asked to indicate whenever a previously seen design is presented. Scores that reflect total correct responses and total correct geometric versus nonsense designs are obtained, as well as a curve of "forgetting" over the seven trials. The test has been used clinically to differentiate brain-damaged patients from normal patients and to lateralize lesions, and in experimental studies of memory processing.[49]

## Tactual Performance Test (TPT) (I)

Reitan[75] incorporated the TPT in his battery. It had initially been adapted by Halstead from Sequin's original 10-piece wooden form board. The blindfolded patient is required to complete the form board first with the dominant hand only, then with the nondominant hand only, and finally with both hands. After completion of the three trials, all test items and the blindfold are removed, and the patient is instructed to draw a picture of the form board with shapes correctly aligned. Scores are obtained for the time required to complete each trial, for each correct shape remembered during the drawing trial, and for each correctly positioned drawn shape. The presumption in the use of this test is that learning takes place over the three direct trials and that nonverbal memory is tapped during the recall phase. Despite its continuing popularity as a part of the Halstead-Reitan battery, there are many reservations regarding its utility, including the neuropsychologically complex nature of the tasks, the time necessary for administration, and the tremendous discomfort and frustration experienced by many patients. The test does not seem cost-effective in terms of the unique data that it might provide.

## Auditory Verbal Learning Test (AVLT)

The AVLT[78] is an easily administered test of immediate verbal memory span. In five administrations of a 15-word list, the test provides a learning curve and documents learning strategies, retroactive and proactive interferences, and confusion or confabulation tendencies. With additional delayed trials (15 minutes, 60 minutes, 24 hours, and so forth), the test also measures retention over time. Rey[78] and others have provided an objective scoring method and normative data drawn from normal and clinical samples. A nonverbal analog in picture form[25] has also been studied. This test is not widely used in clinical batteries, but it would seem to be useful in assessing patients with memory disorders or in the experimental study of memory.

## Bender Gestalt Recall

Incidental visual memory may be assessed by requesting the patient to recall and produce the nine Bender Gestalt designs shortly after completion of the reproduction phase of the test. In contrast to most memory tests, the patient is not told that he or she will be required to recall the designs, thus eliminating the concentration and practice effects that occur when the patient is aware of the "memory" nature of the test. In

186

initial attempts to standardize this procedure, we have found that normal subjects correctly recall a mean of six designs (standard deviation of approximately one). It has been useful in demonstrating defects in patients who perform relatively adequately on the Wechsler Memory Scale or the BVRT when they know that they must make a concentrated effort to remember.

## TESTS OF ABSTRACTION AND HIGHER COGNITIVE PROCEDURES

### Shipley-Hartford Scale (K)

The Shipley-Hartford Scale[81] is a measure of verbal logical reasoning, in which performance on a subtest of verbal abstract reasoning presented as a series of incomplete progressions (e.g., up-down, in-out, come-_) is contrasted with a baseline multiple-choice vocabulary test. The rationale underlying the use of this test is that with many organic deficits, vocabulary will usually be better retained, while abstraction and intellectual efficiency will show greater impairment. Swiercinsky[89] suggested, on the basis of a factor analytic study, that the Shipley was a time- and cost-effective and clinically appropriate substitute for the much more time consuming Category Test for assessing abstraction.

### Wisconsin Card Sorting Test (F)

The Wisconsin Card Sorting Test,[12] which was designed to assess abstract ability, conceptual shifting, and "learning to learn," has recently been restandardized in terms of administration and scoring directions and has been subjected to a more refined standardization study.[39] The test requires the patient to sort a series of printed cards according to color, form, or number, with the corrected category shifting without notice each time the criterion of 10 consecutive correct responses is reached. The patient is told whether a response is right or wrong, but is not informed that the category will shift or what the correct category is. This test has received renewed neuropsychologic attention because: (1) it provides an objective measure of abstraction; (2) it is sensitive to the effects of frontal lobe lesions; and (3) it gives information on the particular reasons for difficulty on the test (e.g., impaired conceptualization, failure to sustain the correct set, perseveration, or deficits in learning across several trials).

## Category Test (I)

The Category Test[76] is considered by many to be among the most sensitive tests of the Halstead-Reitan battery to the effects of brain dysfunction. It is a projector administered measure of abstract reasoning and problem solving, which requires the patient to learn sorting behavior based upon such variables as size, shape, number, color, position, and brightness. Category Test performance is significantly related to age, education, and intelligence, resulting in interpretation problems when evaluating the performance of some patients. The Category Test is expensive, time-consuming, and frustrating to many patients. These logistical problems, combined with the psychologic complexity of the test and the questionable nature of the derived test score, raise a serious question as to the cost, time, validity, and utility of this widely used instrument. In efforts to deal with at least the cost and logistics problems, both short forms[16] and paper-and-pencil forms[2,19] of the test have been developed.

## Raven's Progressive Matrices (G)

The Progressive Matrices[72,73,74] is a test of visual-spatial analysis, spatial conceptualization, and numerical reasoning. The test is available in three difficulty levels, ranging from the Coloured Matrices for children and impaired adults to the Advanced Matrices for well-functioning adults. It is easily administered, taking from 15 to 30 minutes, and requires the patient to select a pictured pattern to best complete a stimulus pattern with an omitted portion. The matrices are useful for assessing visual pattern matching, nonverbal reasoning, unilateral neglect, and cognitive style.

In patients with known perceptual-motor constructional deficits, the test can be useful for differentiating between the visual-spatial analytic and the motor-integration components of the problem. In brain-damaged patients, the degree of impairment seems directly related to the extent of damage, with a tendency for right-hemisphere damaged patients to perform less adequately, especially on the colored version of the test.[76]

## Proverbs Test (H)

A variety of proverb interpretation tests have been devised to assess the patient's level of abstract versus concrete thinking. Verbal abstraction should be considered to be a continuum, ranging from complete abstract thinking to absolute concreteness. Accordingly, the response to proverbs should not be interpreted in a dichotomous fashion (concrete-abstract), but rather by rating the answer on a scale (e.g., 1, 2, 3, 4, 5) that objectifies the degree of abstract ability. The Proverbs Test[33] is a standardized test of proverbs with regard to familiarity and difficulty. The patient is presented with four alternative interpretations for each proverb, one of which is the correct abstract response, one of which is a literal, concrete interpretation, and two of which are either of variable levels of inaccuracy or are common misinterpretations. The structured multiple-choice format of the test has the advantage of providing objective scores of both abstraction and concreteness that can be compared with standard norms. It does not allow the total inadequacy of interpretation or the variety of concrete responses that are produced by some patients on less-structured versions of the task.

## Trail Making Test (I)

This test,[75] which is included in the Halstead-Reitan battery, has enjoyed continued popularity as a measure of visual searching, visual sequencing, perceptual-motor speed, and the ability to make alternating conceptual shifts. It is administered in two parts: Form A requires the patient to draw a line connecting 25 pseudorandomly numbered circles on a standard sheet of paper. Part B requires the patient to alternate between numbers and letters (i.e., 1 – A – 2 – B – 3 . . .) to connect the same number of circles. The patient is instructed to complete the tests "as rapidly but accurately as possible," since the score is the total time required to complete each form. Standard norms for various age groups are available,[18] as are a variety of data from specific clinical samples (e.g., Lewinson[55]). Research has indicated that this test is highly sensitive to the effects of brain dysfunction of any type and provides some indication that patients with frontal lobe lesions perform relatively more poorly.

# TESTS OF PERCEPTUAL FUNCTIONING

## Seashore Rhythm Test (G, I)

This test, which is a part of the Seashore Test of Musical Talent, has also been an integral aspect of the Halstead-Reitan battery[77] and many of its derivatives. It requires the patient to discriminate between pairs of musical tones that are either the same or different. The Rhythm Test is primarily used to assess right temporal lobe functioning, although impaired performance may result from more diffuse lesions.[8]

## Speech Sounds Perception Test (I)

This subtest of the Halstead-Reitan battery[75,76] requires the patient to indicate on an answer sheet which of four nonsense speech-like syllables he or she has heard via tape recorder headphones. The test includes 60 sets of syllables based on the vowel sound "ee" but beginning and ending with different consonants. It is an effective measure of sustained attention and has been consistently reported to be sensitive to the effects of brain damage, particularly left temporal lesions.

## Tests of Tactile Perception

A variety of objective tests of tactile suppression, tactile recognition (stereognosis), and graphasthesia (e.g., fingertip writing, palm writing) have been developed to assess unilateral parietal lobe functioning. With the exception of normative data for objective comparison, they are very similar to the tests conducted during the standard neurologic and extended mental status examinations.

## Tests of Visual Perception

It is crucial to establish the adequacy of the patient's visual acuity and visual perception and to rule out the possibility of unilateral neglect or inattention. Much of this is accomplished using clinical methods akin to the standard neurologic exam. Tests of neglect,[3] color vision,[42] visual recognition,[11] facial recognition,[11] fragmented visual stimuli,[56] and figure-ground discrimination[17,92] are merely examples of the many standardized tests and procedures that can be used to assess these functions. See Lezak[54] for a comprehensive review.

# TESTS OF CONSTRUCTIONAL ABILITY

## Bender-Gestalt Test (G)

The Bender Gestalt Test (originally the Bender Visual Motor Gestalt[7]) is a venerable rapid screening test of paper-and-pencil constructional ability. The patient reproduces each of nine geometric line and dot drawings. The design reproductions can be objectively scored for the errors of integration, distortion, perseveration, and rotation.[50] The designs are sufficiently simple that errorless performance is expected by age 12. The use of this test as a "screen" for organicity, unfortunately still a relatively common practice, is totally unwarranted given the current state of knowledge regarding brain-behavior relationships. However, its inclusion as a test of one type of constructional ability within a more comprehensive battery seems appropriate. It is sensitive to neurologic lesions in virtually all quadrants of the brain, especially in the nondominant hemisphere.[13] Golden[28] provides a thorough review of the advantages and disadvantages of this popular test.

## Raven's Progressive Matrices (G)

See Tests of Abstraction and Higher Cognitive Procedures for a discussion of this test, which is useful in assessing the visual-spatial analytic component of the constructional process.

## Benton Visual Retention Test (G)

See Tests of Memory for a review of this well-standardized test, which can be used to evaluate both reproduction constructional ability (design copying) and short-term recall reproduction (constructions from memory). The major advantages of this test are standard administration and scoring criteria, good normative data, and the availability of alternate equivalent forms.

## Minnesota Perception-Diagnostic Test (K)

This copying test[26] is similar in approach to the Bender Gestalt and Benton Visual Retention Test. The test employs a design copying format, with the reproductions being objectively scored for the degree of rotation. Normative data is provided for both adults and children.

## Additional Tests of Constructional Ability

A wide range of clinical tests of construction have been used to supplement the more objectively scored and normed instruments. These include drawings to command (e.g., human figure drawing, bicycle drawing), geometric block constructions (e.g., WAIS-R Block Designs, Grassi Block Substitution), puzzle completion (e.g., WAIS-R Objective Assembly), and stick and three-dimensional reproductions. See Benton and associates[11] and Lezak[54] for reviews.

# TESTS OF VISUAL SEQUENCING

## Symbol Digit Modalities Test (K)

This test[83] is an analog of the Digit Symbol and Coding subtests of the Wechsler series of intelligence tests, in that the patient is presented with a series of nine symbols, each of which is associated with a number 1 to 9. The patient then places as many numbers with the correct randomly ordered symbols as possible within a 90-second time period. The test can be administered with either a written or verbal response, allowing a comparison of performance in each modality. Normative data is provided for age groups from 18 to 74, and for groups of differing educational levels and clinical diagnoses. The Symbol Digit Modalities Test requires sustained attention, visual searching, visual sequencing, and new-learning ability. The test is sensitive to deficits in any of these functions, as well as to brain dysfunction of many types.

## Trail Making Test (I)

See Tests of Abstraction and Higher Cognitive Procedures for a discussion of this test, which can be considered to assess visual sequencing as well as a number of other neuropsychologic functions.

# TESTS OF LANGUAGE PERFORMANCE

## Peabody Picture Vocabulary Test—Revised (A)

The PPVT-R[23] is an easily administered, recently revised and restandardized test of single-word vocabulary comprehension. It includes two equivalent sets of stimuli plates that contain four pictures. The two associated word lists include 175 words that are ordered in ascending difficulty. The patient indicates which of each set of four pictures is most like the word provided by the examiner. Norms are provided for age groups between 2½ and 41 years. The test is useful for many reasons: (1) It serves as a useful "icebreaker," since its graded format allows success at some level; (2) it provides an assessment of the patient's ability to understand spoken language at its simplest (one word) level; and (3) it gives a general approximation of the patient's level of intellectual functioning because of the relatively high correlation between the PPVT-R and standard adult intelligence tests (0.65 to 0.75). It should be emphasized that this is *not* a test of intelligence; neither current nor premorbid IQ estimates should be made from Peabody performance. It's primary utility is in providing an objective test of single-word receptive vocabulary.

## Token Test

The short version of the Token Test[21] is a well-structured, simply administered test of language comprehension. It utilizes plastic tokens that are manipulated by the patient in response to a series of hierarchically ordered verbal commands (e.g., from "touch a red token" to "after touching the yellow circle, pick up the white square"). The test is designed to objectively test the patient's comprehension at seven levels of difficulty. It is useful in the assessment of the aphasic patient, as well as the patient with comprehension deficits secondary to dementia or other neurologic conditions. A number of versions of the Token Test have been devised and are well reviewed in Lezak.[54]

## Boston Naming Test (D)

The Boston Naming Test[44] is the reciprocal of the PPVT-R in that it requires the patient to name a 60-item series of pictured objects ordered in increasing difficulty from "bed" to "abacus." If the patient is unable to spontaneously name an item, the examiner provides first a categorical (e.g., "it's something to eat") and then a phonemic (e.g., the beginning sound of the target word) cue. The test is basically a test of single-word expressive vocabulary or naming ability. Provisional norms are provided for children, normal adults, and aphasic adults.

## Verbal Fluency Test (E)

A number of standardized tests of verbal fluency are currently available. The two that have proven most effective in our setting are the Controlled Oral Word Association Test (FAS or CFL), adopted from the Multilingual Aphasia Examination,[10] and the Animal Naming Test, adopted from the Boston Diagnostic Aphasia Examination.[32] These tests are discussed in Chapter 5. Both provide normative data to assess the patient's ability to spontaneously produce words under the restrictions of a limited category ("F") and time (60 seconds).

Analogs of this verbal task are available for written language[90] and reading.[6]

## Sentence Repetition (D, E)

The two widely used tests of sentence repetition are the Spreen-Benton Sentence Repetition Test[85] and Sentence Repetition.[10] Both tests evaluate the patient's ability to immediately repeat a series of sentences of increasing length and semantic complexity. Norms are provided for both normal and neurologically impaired adults.

## Comprehensive Aphasia Batteries

When evaluating a patient with known aphasia or a clinically apparent language obstacle to valid neuropsychologic evaluation, a complete aphasia examination should be conducted. In some settings, this is the responsibility of the speech pathologist; in other settings, such batteries are used by the neuropsychologist. In either case, the clinician who deals with brain-damaged patients should be familiar with the contents as well as the advantages and disadvantages of the commonly used tests. The following is an annotated listing of the more popular batteries; the reader is referred to Albert and associates,[4] Lezak,[54] and Kertesz[46] for more thorough reviews of evaluation in aphasia, as well as for the specific tests. Test batteries are listed in alphabetical order without reference to their quality or popularity.

### Aphasia Language Performance Scales (from authors)

This is a short (30 minutes) test[45] of communicative ability designed primarily to determine the suitability of the patient for speech therapy.

### Boston Diagnostic Aphasia Examination (D)

This is a highly clinical battery[32] that systematically assesses virtually all areas of language. The test is useful for the description of aphasic disorders, treatment planning, and research.

### Communication Abilities in Daily Living (University Park Press)

This is a test[41] of functional daily communication ability in aphasic adults, which is primarily used by speech therapists to determine those aspects of communication that should be treated to maximize functional communication.

### Multilingual Aphasia Examination (University of Iowa)

This is a research-derived systematic examination[10] of the major components of speech and language. Each scale is objectively and independently scored, allowing independent use of subtests. The examination is neuropsychologically oriented and appropriate for research.

Neurosensory Center Comprehensive Examination for Aphasia (E)

This is a battery[86] that assesses 20 different components of language. It also includes four tests of tactile and visual functioning. Because of its content, it is useful for neurolinguistic research, but suffers somewhat when used clinically with mild aphasics.

Porch Index of Communicative Ability (B)

The PICA[66] is a highly structured, standardized, psychometrically oriented battery that is used to quantify a variety of communicative functions, including verbal, gestural, and graphic. The test is most frequently used by speech pathologists to establish baseline levels, predict probable recovery, and to quantify the results of therapy and spontaneous improvement. Its statistical sophistication allows certain types of research; however, because it is psychometrically, not clinically, oriented, it is not very useful in the neurobehavioral study of the classic aphasic syndromes.

Western Aphasia Battery (Grune and Stratton)

This battery[47] is essentially an adaptation and standardization of the Boston Diagnostic Aphasia Examination, incorporating many of the same items and utilizing the same theoretical framework for classification of aphasic subtypes. It includes tests of constructional ability, arithmetic, praxis, and Raven's Matrices to assess functions that are related to communication. The test is relatively new, and its clinical and research utility above that of the more established BDAE remains unknown. It is incidentally interesting that the Western Aphasia Battery was designed for and standardized on Canadians.

# TESTS OF MOTOR COORDINATION AND STRENGTH

## Finger Tapping Test (I, J)

The Finger Tapping Test,[75,77] also known as the Finger Oscillation Test, is a frequently used measure of fine motor coordination and speed.

A variety of administration methods have been published, with all involving a number of tapping trials by the index finger of each hand and a recording tapping device. A number of repeats suggest an average of approximately 55 ± 5 taps with the dominant hand during a 10-second trial and approximately 50 ± 4 taps with the nondominant hand. The test is fairly sensitive to brain dysfunction in general and, more specifically, to lesions in the area of the contralateral motor strip.[36]

## Hand Dynamometer (Grip Strength) (I, J)

The use of a mechanical hand dynamometer to assess grip strength with the right and left hands allows the accurate quantification of a common component of the standard neurologic examination. Standard norms are available from the many studies of the Halstead-Reitan battery and other related literature.[89] Reductions in strength bilaterally when compared with the expected levels for age and sex, as well as disproportionate discrepancies between hands, may be indicative of brain dysfunction if peripheral factors are ruled out.

## Miscellaneous Motor Tests

In addition to these routinely administered tests, a wide variety of motor and motor-related instruments are available when more extensive testing of these functions is indicated. Among the more frequently used are the Porteus Maze Test,[67] the Luria Alternating Hand Series,[17] the Purdue Pegboard Test,[93] and the Grooved Pegboard.[61] See Anastasi[5] and Lezak[54] for descriptions of these tests and additional measures.

# TESTS OF ACADEMIC ACHIEVEMENT

## Gates-MacGinitie Reading Tests (Teachers College Press)

The Gates-MacGinitie[27] is a paper-and-pencil, multiple-choice test that assesses various aspects of reading through a grade level of 12. The test is useful when it is necessary or theoretically interesting to examine the reading areas in relative isolation (e.g., reading speed versus comprehension). It may be less useful with educated adults with relatively minor reading problems.

## Peabody Individual Achievement Test (A)

The PIAT[24] measures reading recognition, comprehension, spelling, arithmetic, and general information in children and adults. It uses a

196

multiple-choice format and is particularly useful when assessing the verbal, but physically handicapped, patient. Obviously, it is not valid for evaluating patients with language problems. The test is well standardized and provides norms for age groups between 5.3 and 18.3 years.

## Wide Range Achievement Test (C, G)

The WRAT[43] is probably the most frequently used clinical standard test of achievement, due in part to its brevity. It assesses performance in reading recognition, spelling to dictation, and arithmetic. The test has been recently restandardized and is a useful clinical achievement test for both children and adults. A large-print version of the test protocol is available for use with patients who have visual deficits.

# PERSONALITY TESTS

## Minnesota Multiphasic Personality Inventory (MMPI) (G)

The MMPI[38] continues to be the most commonly used standardized test of emotional status in both psychiatric and neurologic patents. The test consists of 566 statements (e.g., "I am under a great deal of tension") to which the patient responds "true" or "false" as they apply to him or her. The protocol is scored using either a standard or a wide variety of normed templates, with the resultant scores plotted on a graph that shows the patient's performance in the clinical areas of hypochondriasis, depression, hysteria, psychopathic deviance, masculinity-femininity of interests, paranoia, psychasthenia (obsessive-compulsive), schizophrenia, hypomania, and social introversion. Validity scales of L (lie or inconsistency of responses), F (abnormal items suggesting either an attempt to "fake bad" or frank psychopathology), and K (a superior variable reflecting social awareness, defensiveness, and attempts to "fake good") are obtained to help in judging the validity of test behavior. Scores on experimental scales such as "low back pain" or "ego strength" can be plotted in a similar fashion. In general, scores more than two standard deviations above the mean are considered abnormal. A wide variety of interpretive guidebooks are available for general physicians, psychiatrists, and psychologists to aid in understanding the clinical significance of the profile. There has been an increasing interest in the application of computer administration, scoring, and interpretation of this test. At our current state of knowledge, such an approach is more appropriate for normal and mildly abnormal psychiatric patients than for brain-damaged patients. The literature that pertains to the use of the MMPI with brain-damaged patients is expanding, with the reviews by Golden[28,31] and Lezak[54] serving as useful introductions. With some caution, the MMPI appears to provide a reasonably objective picture of the emotional changes seen in neurologic patients.

## Other Personality Instruments

A variety of patient self-reporting scales of anxiety, depression, psychosocial pain, and social adjustment are available for those patients who are capable of responding validly. Such tests may be useful for assessing the subjective perception of emotional and social well-being, as well as for research. See Lezak[54] and Sweetland and Keyser[88] for more information.

# REFERENCES

1. Adams, K. M.: In search of Luria's battery: A false start. J Consult Clin Psychol 48:511–516, 1980.
2. Adams, R. L. and Tranton, S. L.: Development of a paper-and-pen form of the Halstead Category Test. J Consult Clin Psychol 49:298–299, 1981.
3. Albert, M. L.: A simple test of visual neglect. Neurology 23:658, 1973.
4. Albert, M. L., et al: Clinical Aspects of Dysphasia. Springer-Verlag, New York, 1981.
5. Anastasi, A.: Psychological Testing, ed. 5. Macmillan, New York, 1982.
6. Baehr, M. E. and Corsini, R. J.: The Press Test. London House Press, Park Ridge, Ill., 1982.
7. Bender, L.: Bender Motor Gestalt Test. American Orthopsychiatric Association, New York, 1946.
8. Beniak, T. E.: The assessment of cognitive deficits in uremia. Paper presented at the European meeting of the International Neuropsychological Society, Oxford, England, 1977.
9. Benton, A. L.: The Revised Visual Retention Test, ed. 4. Psychological Corporation, New York, 1974.
10. Benton A. L. and Hamsher, K.: Multilingual Aphasia Examination. University of Iowa Press, Iowa City, 1978.
11. Benton, A. L., et al: Contributions to Neuropsychological Assessment: A Clinical Manual. Oxford University Press, New York, 1983.
12. Berg, E. A.: A simple objective technique for measuring flexibility in thinking. J Gen Psychol 39:15–22, 1948.
13. Black, F. W. and Bernard, B.: Constructional apraxia as a function of lesion locus and size in patients with focal brain damage. Cortex 20:111, 1984.
14. Boll, T. J.: The Halstead-Reitan Neuropsychology Battery. In Filskov, S. B. and Boll, T. J. (eds.): Handbook of Clinical Neuropsychology. Wiley-Interscience, New York, 1981, pp. 577-607.
15. Browne, E. R., Randt, C. T., and Osborne, D. P.: Assessment of memory disturbances in aging. In Agnol, et al (eds.): Aging, Vol. 23, Aging Brain and Ergot Alkaloids. Raven Press, New York, 1983, pp. 131-137.

16. Calsyn, D. A., O'Leary, M. R., and Chaney, E. F.: Shortening the Category Test. J Consult Clin Psychol 48:788–789, 1980.
17. Christensen, A. L.: Luria's Neuropsychological Investigation, ed. 2. Munksgaard, Copenhagen, Western Psychological Services, Los Angeles, 1979.
18. Davies, A.: The influence of age on Trail Making Test performance. J Clinical Psychol 24:96, 1968.
19. DeFilippus, N. A. and McCampbell, M. S.: The Booklet Category Test. Psychological Assessment Resources, Odessa, Florida, 1980.
20. Delise, D. C. and Kaplan, E.: Hazards of a standardized neuropsychological test with low content validity: Comment on the Luria-Nebraska Neuropsychological battery. J Consult Clin Psychol 51:396, 1983.
21. DeRenzi, E. and Faglioni, P.: Normative data and screening power of a shortened version of the Token Test. Cortex 14:41, 1978.
22. Dodrill, C. B.: Sex differences on the Halstead-Reitan neuropsychological measures. J Clin Psychol 35:236–241, 1979.
23. Dunn, L. M. and Dunn, L. M.: Peabody Picture Vocabulary Test—Revised. American Guidance Service, Circle Pines, Minnesota, 1981.
24. Dunn, L. M. and Markwardt, F. O.: Peabody Individual Achievement Test. American Guidance Service, Circle Pines, Minnesota, 1970.
25. Fowler, R. S.: A simple non-language test of new learning. Percept Mot Skills 29:895–901, 1969.
26. Fuller, G. B.: Minnesota Perceptuo-Diagnostic Test (Revised Edition). Clinical Psychology Publishing, Brandon, Vermont, 1969.
27. Gates, A. I. and MacGinitie, W. H.: Gates-MacGinitie Reading Tests. Teachers College Press (Columbia), New York, 1969.
28. Golden, C. J.: Clinical interpretation of objective psychological tests. Grune & Stratton, New York, 1979.
29. Golden, C. J.: A standardized version of Luria's neuropsychological tests. In Filskov, S. B. and Boll, T. J. (eds.): Handbook of Clinical Neuropsychology. Wiley-Interscience, New York, 1981, pp. 608–642.
30. Golden, C. J., Hammeke, T. A., and Purisch, A. D.: Manual for the Luria-Nebraska Neuropsychological Battery. Western Psychological Services, Los Angeles, 1980.
31. Golden, C. J. and Vicente, P. J. (eds.): Foundations of Clinical Neuropsychology. Plenum Publishing, New York, 1983.
32. Goodglass, H. and Kaplan, E.: The Assessment of Aphasia and Related Disorders, ed. 2. Lea & Febiger, Philadelphia, 1983.
33. Gorham, D. R.: The Proverbs Test. Psychological Test Specialists, Missoula, Montana, 1956.
34. Grahan, F. K. and Kendall, B. S.: Memory-for-Designs Test: Revised general manual. Percept Mot Skills (Suppl) 2-VIII, 11, 147–188, 1960.
35. Green, R. F. and Martinez, J. N. (translators): Escala de Inteligencia Wechsler para adultos. Psychological Corporation, New York, 1968.
36. Haaland, K. Y. and Delaney, H. D.: Motor deficits after left or right hemisphere damage due to stroke or tumor. Neuropsychologia 19:17, 1981.
37. Halstead, W.: Brain and intelligence: A qualitative study of the frontal lobes. University of Chicago Press, Chicago, 1947.
38. Hathaway, S. R. and McKinley, J. C.: The Minnesota Multiphasic Personality Inventory. Psychological Corporation, New York, 1951.
39. Heaton, R. K: Wisconsin Card Sorting Test Manual. Psychological Assessment Resources, Odessa, Florida, 1981.
40. Heaton, R. K., Baade, L. E., and Johnson, K. L.: Neuropsychological tests results associated with psychiatric disorders in adults. Psychol Bull 85:141–162, 1978.

41. Holland, A. L.: Communicative Abilities in Daily Living. University Park Press, Baltimore, 1980.
42. Ishihara, S.: Tests for Color-blindness. Kanehara Shuppan, Tokyo, 1964.
43. Jastak, S. and Wilkinson, G. S.: The Wide Range Achievement Test (Revised). Jastak Associates, Wilmington, Delaware, 1984.
44. Kaplan, E., Goodglass, H., and Weintraub, S.: Boston Naming Test. Lea & Febiger, Philadelphia, 1983.
45. Keenan, J. S. and Brassell, E. G.: Aphasia Language Performance Scales (ALPS). Pinnacle Press, Murfeesboro, Tenn., 1975.
46. Kertesz, A.: Aphasia and Related Disorders: Taxonomy, Localization, and Recovery. Grune & Stratton, New York, 1979.
47. Kertesz, A.: The Western Aphasia Battery. Grune & Stratton, New York, 1982.
48. Kimura, D.: Right temporal-lobe damage: Perception of unfamiliar stimuli after damage. Arch Neurol 8:264–271, 1963.
49. Kimura, D. and McGlone, J.: Neuropsychology Test Procedures. D. K. Consultants, London, 1983.
50. Koppitz, E. M.: The Bender Gestalt Test for Young Children. Grune & Stratton, New York, 1964.
51. Lawson, J. S., Inglis, J., and Stroud, T. W. F.: A laterality index of cognitive impairment derived from a principal components analysis of the WAIS-R. J Consult Clin Psychol 51:841–847, 1983.
52. Leiter, R. G.: Examiner's Manual for the Leiter International Performance Scale. Stoelting, Chicago, 1969.
53. Leiter, R. G.: General Instructions for the Leiter International Performance Scale. Western Psychological Services, Los Angeles, 1976.
54. Lezak, M. D.: Neuropsychological Assessment. Oxford University Press, New York, 1983.
55. Lewinson, P. M.: Psychological assessment of patients with brain injury. Unpublished Manuscript. University of Oregon, Eugene, Oregon, 1973.
56. Likert, R. and Quasha, W. H.: The Revised Minnesota Paper Form Board Test. Psychological Corporation, New York, 1970.
57. Logue, P. and Wyrick, L.: Initial validation of Russell's revised Wechsler Memory Scale: A comparison of normal aging versus dementia. J Consult Clin Psychol 47:176–178, 1979.
58. Marsh, G. G. and Hirsch, S. H.: Effectiveness of two tests of visual retention. J Clin Psychol 38:115–118, 1982.
59. Matarazzo, J. D.: Wechsler's Measurement and Appraisal of Adult Intelligence, ed. 5. Oxford University Press, New York, 1972.
60. Matthews, C. G.: Neuropsychology practice in a hospital setting. In Filskov, S. B. and Boll, T. J. (eds.): Handbook of Clinical Neuropsychology. Wiley-Interscience, New York, 1981, pp. 645–685.
61. Matthews, C. G. and Klove, H.: Instruction Manual for the Adult Neuropsychology Test Battery. University of Wisconsin Medical School, Maddison, Wisconsin, 1964.
62. Melendez, F.: The Adult Neurospychological Questionnaire (ANQ). Psychological Assessment Resources, Odessa, Florida, 1978.
63. O'Donnell, W. E., DeSoto, C. B., and Reynolds, D. McQ.: Sensitivity and specificity of the Neuropsychological Impairment Scale (NIS). J Clin Psychol 40:553, 1984.
64. O'Donnell, W. E., Reynolds, D. McQ., and DeSoto, C. B.: Validity and reliability of the Neuropsychological Impairment Scale (NIS). J Clin Psychol 40:549, 1984.
65. O'Donnell, W. E. and Reynolds, D. McQ.: Neuropsychological Impairment Scale. Unpublished Manual, Annapolis, Md., 1983.
66. Porch, B. E.: Porch Index of Communicative Ability. Consulting Psychologists Press,

Palo Alto, Calif. 1967.

67. Porteus, S. D.: Porteus Maze Test. Psychological Corporation, New York, 1965.

68. Preston, J.: Neuropsychological Screening Exam. The Wilmington Press, Dallas, 1983.

69. Psychological Assessment Resources: Neuropsychological Status Examination. Psychological Assessment Resources, Odessa, Florida, 1983.

70. Randt, C. T. and Brown, E. R.: Administration Manual: Randt Memory Test. Life Science Associates, Bayport, New York, 1983.

71. Randt, C. T., Brown, E. R., and Osborne, D. P.: A memory test for longitudinal measurement of mild to moderate deficits. Clinical Neuropsychology II 4:184–194, 1980.

72. Raven, J. C.: Guide to the standard Progressive Matrices. H. K. Lewis, London, Psychological Corporation, New York, 1977.

73. Raven, J. C.: Guide to using the coloured progressive matrices. H. K. Lewis, London, Psychological Corporation, New York, 1977.

74. Raven, J. C.: The Advanced Progressive Matrices. H. K. Lewis, London, Psychological Corporation, New York, 1977.

75. Reitan, R.: Investigation of the validity of Halstead's measures of biological intelligence. Archives of Neurology and Psychiatry 48:475, 1955.

76. Reitan, R.: A research program on the psychological effects of brain lesions in human beings. In Ellis, N. (ed.): International Review of Research in Mental Retardation, Vol. 1. Academic Press, New York, pp. 153–218, 1966.

77. Reitan, R. and Davison, L. A.: Clinical Neuropsychology: Current Status and Applications. Hemisphere, New York, 1974.

78. Rey, A.: L'exam clinique en psychologic. Presses Universitairer de France, Paris, 1964.

79. Russell, E. W.: A multiple scoring method for the assessment of complex memory functions. J Consult Clin Psychol 43:800–809, 1975.

80. Russell, E. W., Neuringer, C., and Goldstein, G.: Assessment of Brain Damage: A Neuropsychological Key Approach. Wiley-Interscience, New York, 1970.

81. Shipley, W. C.: Institute of Living Scale. Western Psychological Services, Los Angeles, 1946.

82. Smith, A.: Dominant and nondominant hemispherectomy. In Smith, W. L. (ed.): Drugs, Development and Cerebral Functions. Charles C. Thomas, Springfield, Ill., 1972, pp. 37–68.

83. Smith, A.: Symbol Digit Modalitier Test Manual. Western Psychological Services, Los Angeles, 1973.

84. Spiers, P. A.: The Luria-Nebraska Neuropsychological Battery revisited: A theory in practice or just practicing. J Consult Clin Psychol 50:301–306, 1982.

85. Spreen, O. and Benton, A. L.: Sentence Repetition Test. University of Victoria Neuropsychology Laboratory, Victoria, B. C., 1969.

86. Spreen, O. and Benton, A. L.: Neurosensory Center Comprehensive Examination for Aphasia. University of Victoria Neuropsychology Laboratory, Victoria, B. C., 1969.

87. Stambrook, M.: The Luria-Nebraska Neuropsychological Battery: A promise that may be partly fulfilled. J Clin Neuropsychol 5:247–269, 1983.

88. Sweetland, R. C. and Keyser, D. J. (eds.): Tests. Test Corporation of America, Kansas City, 1983.

89. Swiercinsky, D.: Manual for the Adult Neuropsychological Evaluation. Charles C. Thomas, Springfield, Ill., 1978.

90. Talland, G. A.: Deranged Memory. Academic Press, New York, 1965.

91. Terman, L. M. and Merrill, M. A.: Stanford-Binet Intelligence Scale. Houghton Mifflin, Boston, 1973.

92. Thurstone, L. L.: A Factorial Study of Perception. University of Chicago Press, Chicago, 1944.

93. Tiffin, J.: Purdue Pegboard Test. Science Research Association, Chicago, 1948.
94. Tites, R. L.: Neuropsychological Test Manual. Royal Ottawa Hospital, Ottawa, Ontario, 1977.
95. Wechsler, D.: Wechsler Memory Scale. Psychological Corporation, New York, 1973.
96. Wechsler, D.: Wechsler Intelligence Scale for Children—Revised (WISC-R). Psychological Corporation, New York, 1974.
97. Wechsler, D.: Wechsler Adult Intelligence Scale—Revised (WAIS-R). Psychological Corporation, New York, 1981.

# Mental Status Examination Recording Form

## PATIENT INFORMATION

Patient Name:                          Date:
Address:                               Case #:


Phone:                                 Hospital #:
Date of Birth:                         Place of Birth:
Age:                                   Sex:
Education:
    Highest Level:              Age at Completion:
    Failures or Honors:
Handedness:
    Patient:                    Family:
Occupation:
Medical Diagnosis:

    Onset and Nature:

Hemiplegia:
    (Circle):      None      Recovered      Right      Left

Hemianopia:
    (Circle):      None      Recovered      Right      Left

Neurosurgical Information:


EEG Focus:

CT Scan, Brain Scan, Angiogram, etc.:

(Starred items are essential and should be used with all patients.)
   *I. Behavioral Observations

      *A. History of behavior change, memory difficulties, bizarre behavior, change in work habits, etc.

      *B. Physical Appearance:

      *C. Emotional Status: (confusion, depression, anxiety, lability, etc.)

      D. Frontal Lobe Test Results (See Related Cortical Functions):

      *E. Denial or Neglect:

   *II. Level of Consciousness

      *A. Rate: Alert ____ Lethargic ____ Stupor ____ Coma ____

      *B. Describe stimulus necessary to arouse patient, and record patient's response:

   *III. Attention

      *A. Observation of patient during examination:

**\*B.** Digit Repetition: Repeat digits at a rate of one per second

| Item | Check if Correct |
|------|------------------|
| 3 – 7 | _____ |
| 2 – 4 – 9 | _____ |
| 8 – 5 – 2 – 7 | _____ |
| 2 – 9 – 6 – 8 – 3 | _____ |
| 5 – 7 – 1 – 9 – 4 – 6 | _____ |
| 8 – 1 – 5 – 9 – 3 – 6 – 2 | _____ |
| 3 – 9 – 8 – 2 – 5 – 1 – 4 – 7 | _____ |
| 7 – 2 – 8 – 5 – 4 – 6 – 7 – 3 – 9 | _____ |

**C.** Vigilance: Repeat letters at a rate of one per second. Tell patient to indicate by tapping the table whenever he hears the letter "A."

L T P E A O A I C T D A L A A

A N I A B F S A M R Z E O A D

P A K L A U C J T O E A B A A

Z Y F M U S A H E V A A R A T

1. Errors of Omission: _____

2. Errors of Commission: _____

**D.** Unilateral Inattention:

**\*IV.** Language

   **\*A.** Spontaneous Speech:

      **\*1.** Describe, including fluency, articulation, and presence of paraphasias:

      2. Verbal fluency: Total words: _____

              Total animals: _____

*B. Comprehension:

   *1.  Patient's response to pointing commands:
        Ask patient to point to one, two, three, then four
        room objects or body parts in sequence. Record ade-
        quacy of performance.


   *2.  Patient's response to yes-no questions:
        (e.g., "Is it raining today?" or "Is Grant still presi-
        dent?")


*C. Repetition:

   Tell the patient to repeat each of the following:

   | | Item | Check if Correct |
   |---|---|---|
   | 1. | Ball | _____ |
   | 2. | Help | _____ |
   | 3. | Airplane | _____ |
   | 4. | Hospital | _____ |
   | 5. | Mississippi River | _____ |
   | 6. | The little boy went home | _____ |
   | 7. | We all went over there together | _____ |
   | 8. | The old car wouldn't start on Tuesday morning | _____ |
   | 9. | The short fat boy dropped the china vase | _____ |
   | 10. | Each fight readied the boxer for the championship bout | _____ |

*D. Naming and Word Finding:

   Tell the patient to name the following simple colors and
   objects:

   | | Item | Check if Correct |
   |---|---|---|
   | 1. | Colors | |
   | | a. Red | _____ |
   | | b. Blue | _____ |
   | | c. Yellow | _____ |
   | | d. Pink | _____ |
   | | e. Purple | _____ |

206

2. Body Parts
   f. Eye     _____
   g. Leg     _____
   h. Teeth     _____
   i. Thumb     _____
   j. Knuckles     _____

3. Clothing & Room Objects
   k. Door     _____
   l. Watch     _____
   m. Shoe     _____
   n. Shirt     _____
   o. Ceiling     _____

4. Parts of Objects
   p. Watch Stem (Winder)     _____
   q. Coat Lapel     _____
   r. Watch Crystal     _____
   s. Sole of Shoe     _____
   t. Buckle of Belt     _____

E. Reading:

Describe level of adequacy (words, sentences, paragraphs) and note types of errors:

F. Writing:

Describe level of adequacy and note types of errors:

G. Spelling:

Describe performance to dictation and note errors:

*V. Memory: Most of the following memory tasks evaluate verbal memory. In patients with language disturbance (aphasia), the visual memory tests must be used.

*A. Immediate Recall (Short-Term Memory):

Refer to Digit Repetition in Section III

*B. Orientation:

Check if Correct

*1.  Person
    a.  Name                              _____
    b.  Age                                 _____
    c.  Birthdate                       _____

*2.  Place
    a.  Location (at present)       _____
    b.  City Location               _____
    c.  Home Address             _____

*3.  Time
    a.  Date                            _____
    b.  Day of the Week          _____
    c.  Time of Day               _____
    d.  Season of the Year       _____
    e.  Duration of Time with Examiner    _____

*C. Remote Memory:

Check if Correct
or Adequate

*1.  Personal Information
    a.  Where were you born?      _____
    b.  School Information        _____
    c.  Vocational History         _____
    d.  Family Information         _____

*2.  Historical Facts
    a.  Four Presidents during your
        lifetime                        _____
    b.  Last War                   _____

*D. New-Learning Ability:

Tell the patient, "I am going to tell you four words which I want you to remember." Have the patient repeat the four words after they are initially presented and then tell him that you will ask him to remember the words later. Continue with the examination, and at intervals of 5, 10, and 30 minutes, ask him to recall the words. Use categorical ("one word is a color") or phonemic ("one word begins with B") cues if he is unable to spontaneously recall the word on any trial.

Record the type and amount of cuing necessary. Two alternate sets of words are provided.

1.    Four Unrelated Words    5 min.  10 min.  30 min.

    a.  Brown      (Fun)      _____   _____   _____
    b.  Honesty    (Loyalty)  _____   _____   _____
    c.  Tulip      (Carrot)   _____   _____   _____
    d.  Eyedropper (Ankle)    _____   _____   _____

Describe type of cues used if necessary:

2.    Verbal Story For Immediate Recall:
      Tell the patient, "I am going to read you a short story which I want you to remember. Listen closely to what I read because I will ask you to tell me the story when I finish." Read the story slowly and carefully, but without pausing at the slash marks. After completing the paragraph, tell the patient to retell the story as accurately as possible. Record the number of correct memories (information within the slashes) and describe confabulation if it is present.

It was July/ and the Rogers/ had packed up/ their four children/ in the station wagon/ and were off/ on vacation.

They were taking/ their yearly trip/ to the beach/ at Gulf Shores.

This year/ they were making/ a special/ two day stop/ at the World's Fair/ in New Orleans.

After a long day's drive/ they arrived/ at the motel/ only to discover/ that in their excitement/ they had left/ the twins/ and their suitcases/ in the front yard.

    a.  Number of correct memories: _____
    b.  Describe confabulation if present:

3.    Visual Memory (Hidden Objects):
      Tell the patient that you are going to hide some

objects around the office, desk, or bed and that you want him to remember where they are. Hide 4 or 5 common objects (keys, pen, reflex hammer, etc.) in various areas in the patient's sight. After a delay of several minutes, ask the patient to find the objects. Ask him to name those items he is unable to find.

a. Number of hidden objects found: _____
b. Number of hidden objects named but not found: _____
c. Number of locations indicated but objects not named: _____

4. Visual Memory (Visual Design Reproduction):
(See Stimulus Cards)

| Item | Score |
|---|---|
| a. Design 1 | _____ |
| b. Design 2 | _____ |
| c. Design 3 | _____ |
| d. Design 4 | _____ |

Total Score _____

5. Paired Associate Learning:
Tell the patient that you are going to read a list of words two at a time. He will be expected to remember the words that go together (e.g., big—little). When he is clear as to the directions, read the first list of words at the rate of one pair per second. After reading the first list, test for recall by presenting the first recall list. Give the first word of a pair and ask for the word that went with it. Correct incorrect responses and proceed to the next pair. After the first recall has been completed, allow a 10-second delay and continue with the second presentation and recall lists.

Presentation Lists

| 1 | 2 |
|---|---|
| a. Weather—Bag | a. House—Income |
| b. High—Low | b. Weather—Bag |
| c. House—Income | c. Book—Page |
| d. Book—Page | d. High—Low |

## Recall Lists

| | 1 | | 2 |
|---|---|---|---|
| a. | House _____ | a. | High _____ |
| b. | High _____ | b. | House _____ |
| c. | Weather _____ | c. | Book _____ |
| d. | Book _____ | d. | Weather _____ |

      1. Number of easy paired associates recalled: _____

      2. Number of difficult paired associates recalled: _____

## *VI. Constructional Ability

### *A. Reproduction Drawings:
Ask the patient to copy the following drawings in the space provided.

|  | Item | Score |
|---|---|---|
| 1. | Vertical Diamond | _____ |
| 2. | Two-Dimensional Cross | _____ |
| 3. | Three-Dimensional Cube | _____ |
| 4. | Three-Dimensional Pipe | _____ |
| 5. | Triangle within a Triangle | _____ |

Total Score: _____

*B. Drawings to Command:
   Tell the patient to draw the following pictures in the space provided.

   Clock with all numbers

   Daisy in flowerpot

   House in Perspective

|  | Item | Score |
|---|---|---|
| 1. | Clock | _____ |
| 2. | Daisy in Flowerpot | _____ |
| 3. | House in Perspective | _____ |

Total Score: _____

C. Block Designs:
  (See Stimulus Cards)

|  | Item | Score |
|---|---|---|
| 1. | Design 1 | _____ |
| 2. | Design 2 | _____ |
| 3. | Design 3 | _____ |
| 4. | Design 4 | _____ |

Total Score: _____

Describe types of errors:

*VII. Higher Cognitive Functions

A. Fund of Information:

|  | Item | Check if Correct |
|---|---|---|
| 1. | How many weeks are in a year? | _____ |
| 2. | Why do people have lungs? | _____ |
| 3. | Name four presidents since 1940. | _____ |
| 4. | Where is Denmark? | _____ |
| 5. | How far is it from New York to Los Angeles? | _____ |
| 6. | Why are light colored clothes cooler in the summer than dark colored clothes? | _____ |
| 7. | What is the capital of Spain? | _____ |
| 8. | What causes rust? | _____ |
| 9. | Who wrote the Odyssey? | _____ |
| 10. | What is the Acropolis? | _____ |

Total Score: _____

*B. Calculations:
Describe the patient's adequacy in performance and types of errors made on the following types of calculations:

1. Verbal Rote Examples:
   a. Addition          ( 4 + 6 )
   b. Subtraction       ( 8 − 5 )
   c. Multiplication    ( 2 × 8 )
   d. Division          ( 56 ÷ 8 )

2. Verbal Complex Examples:
   a. Addition          ( 14 + 17)
   b. Subtraction       ( 43 − 38)
   c. Multiplication    ( 21 × 5)
   d. Division          (128 ÷ 8)

*3. Written Complex Examples:
   a. Addition                          108
                                      + 79

   b. Subtraction                       605
                                      − 86

   c. Multiplication                    108
                                      × 36

   d. Division                       43 / 559

*C. Proverb Interpretation:
Tell the patient to explain the following sayings. Record the answers.

| | Item | Score |
|---|---|---|
| 1. | Don't cry over spilled milk. | _____ |
| 2. | Rome wasn't built in a day. | _____ |
| 3. | A drowning man will clutch at a straw. | _____ |
| 4. | A golden hammer breaks an iron door. | _____ |
| 5. | The hot coal burns; the cold one blackens. | _____ |

Total Score: _____
Total Concrete Responses: _____

*D. Similarities

| | Item | Score |
|---|---|---|
| 1. | Turnip ....... Cauliflower | _____ |
| 2. | Car .......... Airplane | _____ |
| 3. | Desk ........ Bookcase | _____ |
| 4. | Poem ........ Novel | _____ |
| 5. | Horse ........ Apple | _____ |

Total Score: _____
Total Concrete Responses: _____

E. Conceptual Series Completion:

|  | Item | Check if Correct |
|---|---|---|
| 1. | A  B  C  D ___ | _____ |
| 2. | 1  4  7  10 ___  ___ | _____ |
| 3. | AZ  BY  CX  D ___ | _____ |
| 4. | tote to snow on spun up stab ___  ___ | _____ |
| 5. | elephant 87654321 plan 5732 lap ___  ___  ___ | _____ |

Total Score: _____

## VIII. Related Cortical Functions

A. Ideomotor Apraxia:
Describe the adequacy of the patient's performance in carrying out motor acts to command using buccofacial, limb, and whole body commands. Indicate if imitation or use of the real object was necessary to facilitate performance.

|  | Item | Score |
|---|---|---|
| 1. | Blow out a match. | _____ |
| 2. | Drink through a straw. | _____ |
| 3. | Lick crumbs off your lips. | _____ |
| 4. | Comb your hair. | _____ |
| 5. | Flip a coin. | _____ |

B. Ideational Apraxia:
Describe the adequacy of the patient's performance on the following complex motor tasks:

1. Letter-Envelope-Stamp
2. Candle-Holder-Match
3. Toothpaste-Toothbrush

C. Right-Left Disorientation:

|  | Item | Check if Correct |
|---|---|---|
| 1. | Identification on Self | |
| | a.  Show me your right foot | _____ |
| | b.  Show me your left hand | _____ |

2. Crossed Commands on Self

    a. With your right hand touch your left shoulder     _____

    b. With your left hand touch your right ear     _____

3. Identification on Examiner

    a. Point to my left knee     _____

    b. Point to my right elbow     _____

4. Crossed Commands on Examiner

    a. With your right hand point to my left eye     _____

    b. With your left hand point to my left foot     _____

Describe nature and degree of errors made:

D. Finger Agnosia:
Describe the adequacy of the patient's nonverbal and verbal performance.

E. Gerstmann's Syndrome:
Describe the nature and degree of impairment in the following areas if present in the patient:

1. Finger Agnosia:     _____
2. Right-Left Disorientation:     _____
3. Dysgraphia:     _____
4. Dyscalculia:     _____

F. Visual Agnosia:
Describe any deficits in visual identification of objects, naming of objects whose use can be demonstrated, color naming, and facial recognition:

G. Astereognosis:
Describe deficits:

Left hand _____
Right hand _____


H. Geographic Disorientation:

1.  Describe evidence of disorientation obtained from history:


2.  Map Localization:

    Describe patient's ability to localize well-known cities on a map:


3.  Orientation of Self in Hospital:

    Describe patient's ability to orient self within the hospital environment:


*I. Denial and Neglect
If present, describe patient's response

|  | | YES | NO |
|---|---|---|---|
| 1. | Does patient frankly deny his illness? | _____ | _____ |
| 2. | Is there evidence of unilateral neglect? (e.g., shaving one side of face, dressing one arm, etc.) | _____ | _____ |
| 3. | Is there evidence of unilateral neglect on drawings? (e.g., absence of numbers on one side of clock or absence of one side of picture) | _____ | _____ |

J. Frontal Lobe Tests

    1.    Drawings

Tell the patient to copy and continue the following sequence. Record evidence of perseveration or loss of sequence.

    2.    Alternating hand sequences

This is a motor alternation task that utilizes both hands. Initially, the patient places both hands on the desk, one in a fist and one with the fingers extended palm down. Tell the patient to rapidly alternate the position of the two hands (simultaneously extending the fingers of one hand while making a fist with the other). Record if the patient is unable to maintain the alternating sequence.

# SUMMARY OF FINDINGS

1. Describe major areas of impairment:

2. Tentative neurobehavioral diagnosis:

3. Tentative localization:

4. Tentative clinical diagnosis:

5. Proposed management plans:

# Index

A "t" following a page number indicates a table. A page number in *italics* indicates a figure.

Aphasia—*Continued*
  anomic, 172
  defined, 50
  developmental, 50
  digit repetition test and, 42, 43
  dyscalculia accompanying, 135
  emotional reactions to, 174
  finger agnosia seen in patients with, 148
  Gerstmann's syndrome and, 148
  global, 60, 173
  ideomotor apraxia and, 142
  in left-handed persons, 66
  in right-handed persons, 59
  indicating left-hemisphere disease, 158
  language production in, 52
  object naming ability in, 56
  prognosis for aphasia with mild to moderate comprehension defects, 172
  repetition in, 55
  Wernicke's, 61-62, 160, 173
Aphasia Language Performance Scales, 194
Aphasia syndromes, 59, *60*
  anomic, 62, 63-64
  Broca's, 60-61, 63
  conduction, 61-63, *63*
  global, 60
  in left-handed persons, 66
  subcortical, 66
  transcortical, 64-65, *65*, 66
  Wernicke's, 61-62
Aphasia tests, 194-195
Aphasic patients
  ability to perform in verbal learning tasks, 97
  agraphia in, 69
  apraxia in, 55
  evaluation by speech pathologist, 171
  long-term care for, 175
  performance on right-left commands and, 147
  presence of agraphia in, 57
  referral to speech pathologist, 169-170
  visual memory testing and, 84
  writing ability of, 57-58
Aphonia, 73
  hysterical, 170
Apperceptive visual agnosia, 149
Approximate answers syndrome, 98-99
Apraxia, 50, 51
  aphasic patients with, 55
  buccofacial, 50, 51, 140
  defined, 102, 139
  finger agnosia seen in patients with, 148
  ideomotor, 139-144, *143*, *144*
  limb, 102, 140, 143
  limb-kinetic, 139
  of whole body movements, 140

oral, 172, 173
  speech pathologist's role in, 169-170, 171
Apraxic movements, 140-142
Arousal, ascending activating system and, 33. *See also* Consciousness levels
Articulation disturbances, 67-68, 171
  prognosis for, 172
Ascending activating system, 33, 35
  and alterations in level of consciousness, 45
Associative visual agnosia, 149
Astereognosis, 150
Atrophic dementia, 66, 156
Attention
  anatomy and clinical implications of, 44-46
  assessment of, 41-49
  defined, 41
  evaluation of, 42-44
  functional mood alterations affecting, 46
  vs. alertness, 41
Attention disorders, memory testing of patients with, 80
Attentive patient, vs. alert patient, 41
Auditory comprehension, Wernicke's aphasia and, 61-62
Auditory gnosis, 67
Auditory hallucinations, 16
Auditory Verbal Learning Test, 186
Awareness, appearance of, and coma-like states, 35

BACKWARD digit repetition, 80
Basal-orbital lesions in frontal lobe syndrome, 17
Behavior modification techniques, 176
Behavioral observations
  clinical syndromes and, 15-26
  importance of, 12
  mental status examination and, 12-26
  mood and general emotional status of patient, 13-14
  physical appearance and, 12-13
Bender Gestalt Recall Test, 186-187
Bender Gestalt Test, 165, 190-191
Benton Visual Retention Test (BVRT), 185, 191
Bilateral cortical disease
  constructional impairment and, 121
  impairment of higher cognitive functions and, 135
Bilateral lesions located in limbic structures, memory loss and, 96
Bizarre language output, 70, 71-72
Block designs test, 102, 113, *117*, *118*, 119, 120
Bodily cleanliness, lack of attention to, 12, 13

reliability of, 4

sample recording form for, 203–221

shortening of, for patients suspected of dementia, 156

summarizing and organizing data on, 159–160

summary of, 155–160

used for diagnosing organic disease, 6

Metabolic encephalopathy, 15

Midbrain lesion, 35

Mini-mental state test, 159

Minnesota Multiphasic Personality Inventory (MMPI) Test, 197–198

Minnesota Perception-Diagnostic Test, 191

Misalignment in writing, 58

Mood and general emotional status of patient, 13–14

Mood-elevating drugs, 175

Motor activity, behavioral observation of patient and, 13

Motor commands, used in comprehension assessment, 55

Motor coordination and strength tests, 195–197

Multilingual Aphasia Examination Test, 194–195

Multiple sclerosis, 175

Mutism, elective, 73, 170

Myasthenia gravis, 175

NAMING objects, 50, 56, 57t, 71–72

Neglect of one side of body, 22–23, *24*

inattention and, 41

when both sides are simultaneously stimulated, 23

Neologisms

defined, 14

in schizophrenic patients, 70

Neologistic paraphasia, 52

Neuroanatomic lesions, specific language syndromes and, 49

Neurobehavioral diagnosis process on mental status examination, 160

Neurobehavioral disorders, 1, 2

Neurodiagnostic procedures, 3

Neurologists, 169

Neuropsychologic batteries, 181–182

Neuropsychologic evaluation, 3, 163–165

advantages of, 164

clinical services provided by, 167–169

components of, 168

conclusions, 169

referrals, 165–167

vs. mental status examination, 164

Neuropsychologic tests, 179

abstraction and higher cognitive procedures, 125–135, 187–189

academic achievement, 196–197

constructional ability, 102–103, 190–191

intelligence, 182–183

language performance, 50–58, 192–195

memory, 79–92 183–187

motor coordination and strength, 20, 195–196

perceptual functioning, 85–91, 189–190

personality, 197–198

publishers and distributors of, 179–180

screening, 180–182

visual sequencing, 192

Neuropsychological Impairment Scale, 180–181

Neuropsychological Screening Exam, 180, 181

Neuropsychological Status Examination 180, 181

Neuropsychologist

consultations with, 6

qualifications of, 163

role of, in evaluating patients with organic brain disease, 163

Neurosensory Center Comprehensive Examination for Aphasia, 195

Neurotic symptoms, indications of, 14

New-learning ability assessment, 82–83

four unrelated words test, 83

paired associate learning test, 91–92

verbal story for immediate recall test, 84

visual memory (hidden objects) test, 84–85

visual memory (visual design reproduction) test 85–91, *86–90*

Nominal aphasia. *See* Anomic aphasia

Nondominant-hemisphere lesions, 158

as frequent cause of denial and neglect syndrome, 23

Nonfluent aphasia, 52, 53

Nonfluent output, 52. *See also* Aphasia

Nonorganic speech and language disorders, 72–73

Nonverbal memory tasks used for aphasic patients, 97

Nursing home placement, 176

OBJECT agnosia, in patients with ideational apraxia, 145

Obsessive-compulsive neurosis, extreme fastidiousness and, 12, 13

Obtundation, 29, 30

recording degree of, 31, 33t

Ocular motility problems, reading ability testing and, 57

Oral apraxia, 50

prognosis for, 172, 173

Organic affective syndrome, 9

Organic amnesic state, 94–95

memory loss in, 95–96

Organic behavioral change, denial, 22
Organic brain damage, errors on constructional tests indicative of, 117
Organic brain disease
    coexisting with mental illness, 173–175
    consciousness level alterations and, 16
    constructional tasks used in testing for, 101, 102–119, *106–112, 114–118*
    emotional and behavioral changes in, 3
    memory disturbances in, 77
    overlap between symptomatology of emotional disorders and, 9–10
    psychiatric disorders vs., 4, 5, 6
Organic delusional syndrome, 9
Organic disorders, vs. functional disorders, 12, 16
Organic driveness, 45
Organic personality syndrome, 9
"Organic signs," 165
Organic unilateral neglect, 12
Orientation to place and time, assessment of, 81, 93t

Paired Associate Learning (PAL) Test, 91–92, 93t
PAL Test, 91–92, 93t
Panencephalitis, higher cognitive function deficits seen in patients with, 136
Paper-and-pencil reproduction of geometric shapes test, 102. *See also* Reproduction drawings test
Paralexic errors, 57
Paramnesia, 22
Paranoia, 9
    as response to brain damage, 174
Paranoid delusions, 70
Paraphasias, 52
Paresis, 19
Parietal lobe disease, geographic disorientation and, 152
Parietal lobe dysfunction, 120–121
Parietal lobes, 117, 120
Parieto-occipital lesions, finger agnosia and, 148
Parkinsonism, 175
Patient history and mental status examination, 9–12
Patient history outline, 10–12
Patient's medical status, establishment of, before mental status examination, 10
Patient's mental status, use of multiple medications and, 10
Peabody Individual Achievement Test, 196–197
Peabody Picture Vocabulary Test—Revised, 192–193

Perceptual functioning tests, 189–190
Perseveration, 136
Persistent vegetative state, 36
    diagnostic features of, 38t
Personal cleanliness, lack of attention to, 12, 13
Personality disorders, 9. *See also* Organic personality syndrome
Personality tests, 197–198
Phonemic paraphasia, 52
Physical appearance of patients, 12–13
Pick's disease, 19
    remote memory loss in, 98
Pointing commands, used for comprehension assessment, 54
Porch Index of Communicative Ability, 195
Posterior language area, 59, *60*
Postneurosurgical testing, 166
Postoperative period, confusional state in, 16
Post-traumatic amnesia, 79
Posturing of patient, behavioral observation and, 13
Praxis
    defined, 101
    disturbance in, 102
    in left hand, 142
    in right hand, 142
Praxis evaluation, commands used for, 140–142
Premorbid behavior and level of functioning, establishment of, before mental status examination, 10
Preneurosurgical testing, 166
Primary organic brain disease, 2
Problem solving, 126
Prosopagnosia, 149–150
Proverb interpretation, 126, 129, 130–131
Proverbs Test, 188–189
Pseudodementia, 4, 9–10
    defined, 25
    in elderly depressed patient, 26
    vs. early dementia, 26
Psychiatric depressive illness, apathy and psychomotor slowing in patients with, 23
Psychiatric disorders, organic brain disease vs., 4, 5
Psychiatric evaluation, 175
Psychiatric patients
    cognitive deficits on mental status examination and, 10
    use of mental status examination routinely on, 3
Psychiatric treatment, 175–176
Psychiatrist
    reasons for referral of patients to, 173–175

role in rehabilitation of patients with organic brain disease, 173–176
Psychogenic amnesia, 79
memory disturbances in, 98
Psychogenic unresponsiveness, dangers of hasty diagnosis of, 37
Psychologic reports, provided by non-neuropsychologists, 164–165
Psychomotor retardation, 23
Psychomotor slowing, 23
Psychotherapeutic methods, used for patients with organic brain disease, 175
Psychotic language, 70, 71–72
Pure alexia without agraphia, 68
Pure word deafness, 67, 69

QUESTIONS requiring "yes" or "no" answers, used for comprehension assessment, 54–55

RANDOM letter test, 43, 46
Randt Memory Test, 184–185
Raven's Progressive Matrices, 188, 191
Reactive depression, 173
Reading ability
assessment of, 50, 56–57
loss of, 50. *See also* Alexia
Reading comprehension testing, 57
Reading deficit, 56. *See also* Alexia
Reality testing, 14
Recent memory, 78, 94–97
Recent memory, orientation to place and time and, 81
Receptive aphasia, 59
Reciprocal Coordination Test, 20, 22
Recurring Figures Test, 185
Reduplication of body parts, 22
Remote memory, 78, 81, 93t, 97–98
Repetition in speech, 50, 55
impairment in Wernicke's aphasia, 61–62
Reproduction drawings test, 103–105, *104, 106–111*
Responsiveness scale, 31, 33t
Reticular stimulation, 33
Reticular system, damage to extension of brain stem, 35
Retrograde amnesia, 79, 94
Right-handedness, 51, 59
agraphia and, 158
alexia and, 68, 158
aphasia and, 59, 158
Right-hemisphere lesions
apathy seen in patients with, 23
attention and, 46
Right-left disorientation
clinical implications of, 147
evaluation of, 146–147

finger agnosia seen in patients with, 148
Gerstmann's syndrome and, 148
Right-left orientation, 146
Russell Revision of the Wechsler Memory Scale, 184

SCHIZOPHRENIA, 9, 70, 71, 72. *See also* Organic delusional syndrome
diagnosing dementia from, 72
impaired abstracting ability and, 136
Screening tests, 180–182
Seashore Rhythm Test, 189
Semantic paraphasia, 52
Semicoma, 29
Sensory aphasia, 65
Sensory modality, 78
Sentence Repetition Test, 194
Septal rage, 36
Serial sevens subtraction test, 43
Shipley-Hartford Scale, 187
Short-term memory, 78, 80, 198
Similarities test, 132–133
Sleep, as natural fluctuation in level of consciousness, 37
Social awareness, as higher cognitive function, 126, 136
Social judgment, as higher cognitive function, 126, 136
Somnolence, 29. *See also* Lethargy
Spatial analysis tasks, 102
Speech disorder assessment, 14
Speech disorders, requiring evaluation by speech pathologist, 170–171
Speech evaluation, 171–172
Speech melody, 50. *See also* Dysprosody
Speech output, 51
Speech pathologist
as part of rehabilitation team, 168
consultations with, 6
qualifications of, 170
reasons for referring patients to, 170–171
Speech Sounds Perception Test, 190
Spelling ability, 58
Spontaneous drawings test, 102
Spontaneous speech, 50, 51–53
in global aphasia, 60
Stanford-Binet Test, 182–183
Stereognosis, 150
Stick-pattern reproduction test, 102. *See also* Reproduction drawings test
Stimulation responses, levels of consciousness and, 30–33
Store of knowledge, as higher cognitive function, 125. *See also* Fund of information
Stupor, 29
recording degree of, 31, 33t
Stuttering, 171

231